Shoulder Pain

Filip Struyf

Shoulder Pain

Clinical Assessment of a Complex Joint

Springer

Filip Struyf
Department of Rehabilitation
Sciences and Physiotherapy
University of Antwerp
Wilrijk, Belgium

ISBN 978-3-031-82230-8 ISBN 978-3-031-82228-5 (eBook)
https://doi.org/10.1007/978-3-031-82228-5

This Springer imprint is published by the registered company Springer Nature Switzerland AG
The registered company address is: Gewerbestrasse 11, 6330 Cham, Switzerland

Preface

For more than two decades, I have immersed myself in unraveling the mysteries nestled within our shoulders. Ironically, the term "shoulder complex" perfectly captures its intricacy. The shoulder, composed of interconnected joints and bone structures, operates as a harmonious system to execute specific tasks. Typically, these involve positioning our hands—whether bringing food to our mouths, discarding items, retrieving something from a shelf, or opening a door. Our hands are linked to our torsos through the elbow and further to the shoulder. Therefore, the shoulder plays a crucial role in enabling our hands to perform their functions in the right place and at the right time.

As you hold this book, imagine your hand, elbow, shoulder, and even your entire body maintaining equilibrium under the weight of the book. Muscles around your shoulder work to stabilize your upper arm, allowing the elbow to position your hand correctly and keeping the book at the appropriate height and distance from your eyes. In essence, the shoulder enables you to fully enjoy the book—how fitting. In other words, our shoulders are integral to our daily lives, providing a stable foundation for handshakes and requiring the necessary mobility to throw a ball or wave to a neighbor.

Our shoulder serves as the link between the hand and torso, directed by our brains. While our entire body is undoubtedly complex, it is the combination of stability, mobility, and the substantial force our shoulders can generate that renders them unique and complex. Furthermore, even our hormonal and metabolic systems impact how our shoulders feel.

Much of our knowledge about the shoulder has been challenged in the last two decades. The mechanism behind the most common shoulder disorder, shoulder impingement syndrome, is under thorough scrutiny. Treating patients with shoulder instability extends beyond simply contracting muscles around the shoulder, and a frozen shoulder is being reconsidered from a new perspective. More than ever, the biopsychosocial model takes precedence: our body, our thoughts, and our societal well-being matter. This is not a mere castle in the air but a foundation to build upon. Effective communication is crucial in your interaction with a patient experiencing shoulder pain, serving as the cornerstone for understanding, trust, and collaborative decision-making—all of which are immensely important.

Amidst this complexity, with scientific research proliferating, we found ourselves slowly losing sight of the forest for the trees. The simplicity of the previous century turned into a complex entanglement, leading us to believe that only a super-brain could say something meaningful about shoulder function. Due to its complexity, we sometimes overlook the essence, causing both patients and healthcare providers to hesitate out of fear of making a mistake. It is time to zoom out and describe how the cookie crumbles, or in this case, how the upper arm fits into its socket.

I must acknowledge that truth is not absolute. The information in this book may not be exhaustive and may need adjustment with evolving insights. Therefore, it is advisable to verify this information using additional sources before drawing conclusions or making decisions. The ultimate responsibility for clinical decision-making still rests with the clinician and not with a book or other sources of information.

This book is intended as a valuable resource to aid in further developing your expertise and better assisting your patients. Let the insights and information shared herein inspire and empower you to confidently tackle the challenges in shoulder assessment. Together, we are building a future where patient care always takes precedence.

Enjoy reading!

Wilrijk, Belgium
October 2024

Filip Struyf

Acknowledgments

To the healthcare professionals, including students, who have taken this book into their hands, I want to express my deepest gratitude and appreciation. By seeking to expand your knowledge about the shoulder, you demonstrate an unwavering commitment to providing the best possible care for your patients. I wrote this book primarily for you, the dedicated healthcare worker eager to learn more about this remarkable joint, so you can assist your patients even better. I sincerely hope this book broadens your understanding, allowing you to approach shoulder issues with a renewed perspective.

This book reflects my dedication and passion for unraveling the mysteries of the shoulder. It is an honor to share my knowledge and insights with you. Writing this book has been a personal journey through the clinical presentations of patients with shoulder pain. However, this endeavor would not have been possible without the support of many individuals.

I would like to extend my heartfelt thanks to a few key people:

I want to thank Michelle Schellekens for her assistance in transforming the Dutch version of this book into English. I also extend my gratitude to Eoin ó Conaire for his contributions in adding the shoulder assessment framework, which enriches the content significantly.

I would also like to thank Sophie Vanluchene and Sam De Graeve, who modeled for the photos in this book. Your willingness to participate and your contributions to this project are greatly appreciated. Additionally, my sincere thanks go to photographer Pelle De Brabander for his excellent work in capturing the images. I am also incredibly grateful to Lies Poignie and Freya Maenhout from Owl Press for believing in this project and giving me the opportunity to share my knowledge and insights with the world. Their professional guidance, editorial expertise, and unwavering dedication have shaped this book into what it is today. Thanks to their efforts, healthcare professionals worldwide can benefit from this information and better support their patients. In addition, I would like to express my deepest gratitude to the publisher, Springer-Nature, for their belief in me and for agreeing to publish the Dutch version of this book in English. Your support has made this journey possible.

Furthermore, I want to thank all the clinicians and researchers who assisted me in researching and writing this book. Your practical knowledge, experience, and the literature you provided helped me present the content as accurately as possible.

I also want to express my gratitude to the University of Antwerp and FWO (Fonds Wetenschappelijk Onderzoek) for providing me with the space in my schedule to write this book. Your support has been instrumental in making this project a reality.

Finally, my deepest thanks also go to my family and friends, whose unwavering support inspired me and provided the strength to continue, even in the most challenging moments.

Filip Struyf

Disclaimer

In this book, I aim to make existing scientific findings on the clinical assessment of the shoulder accessible. I translate them into an accessible handbook with practical tips. The book covers general information that is not specifically tailored to an individual patient or a particular medical situation. I'm a physical therapist and researcher; I do not provide medical advice but primarily address healthcare providers. The information in this book is not intended as a substitute for services or information from trained (medical) professionals and is certainly not intended as a tool for self-diagnosis.

Introduction

Shoulder pain and impairments are common and a typical reason for a visit to the primary care physician or specialist. Shoulder pain significantly affects the patient's daily life, hobbies, work, and sleep. Historically, the shoulder is viewed as a crucial link in human evolution. We may primarily think of grasping or hanging, but this also pertains to our throwing ability. The prominent journal *Nature* published research comparing the throwing ability of primates, including chimpanzees, with that of humans [1]. One of the most remarkable conclusions was that, thanks to certain anatomical features enabling elastic energy storage in the shoulder, humans have developed an enormous ability to throw at very high speeds. Did you know that we can throw a ball up to 100 miles/h? The researchers further suggest that our development of throwing as a means of hunting likely played a crucial role in our species' evolution. One could almost argue that it is thanks to the evolution of the shoulder that our species still roams this planet. Logically, one might respond that our brains probably played an equally important role. After all, who other than our brains would ensure that the successful throwing technique is programmed into our minds? And who crafted the spear to hit the prey? Fortunately, we need not start a debate on this, but it anecdotally illustrates how important both elements are for the optimal functioning of our shoulder: our brains and our shoulder. Without an anatomically healthy shoulder, we could not hunt, but likewise, without the guiding brain, we could not either. We sometimes describe this as the two wings of a bird. Without both wings, there is no flight. Our shoulders operate in a similar manner. Additionally, we must mention that when we throw a ball at 100 miles/h, this happens not only due to the energy storage in our shoulder. Our torso and lower limbs contribute equally to the entire throwing motion. Therefore, the shoulder must keep the feet on the ground.

Our shoulder functions only when there is a harmonious interplay of various bone structures. But what if a shoulder doesn't function as it should? This can be due to pain, but it can also be a restriction in movement or an unstable feeling in the shoulder. Shoulder pain can start suddenly or worsen gradually. The shoulder may hurt when trying to take something from a cabinet, or even when sitting still in a chair. Sometimes, the patient specifically points out where the pain is, but just as often, the pain extends across the entire shoulder, even reaching the neck, forearm, and hand.

Although research has advanced, the explanation for the cause of pain symptoms is often still unclear. The shoulder's high degree of complexity and the potential mismatch between the injury and pain perception contribute to the ambiguity in the shoulder world. Nevertheless, progress has been made at various levels regarding the scientific background of different shoulder conditions, and uncertainties are giving way to opportunities in treating shoulder pain.

Given the multitude of tests available to examine the shoulder and the variety of conditions, it is essential to proceed methodically. The clinical examination should inform us about the patient's possible condition, specifically identifying anatomical disorders, functional impairments, activity limitations, participation problems, factors that inhibite recovery, and factors that promote recovery. The more precise the location, nature, and manifestation of the injury, the more precise the treatment goals and plans can be developed, catering to the patient's needs. Throughout this process, effective communication forms the essential foundation, where possessing the necessary knowledge alone is not sufficient. We must convey this knowledge in a meaningful, respectful, sensitive, and effective manner. Listening to the personal story is crucial for healthcare providers as it enables us to tailor our communication to individual needs. Communication permeates every aspect of healthcare, involving building relationships, creating trust, and forging a strong therapeutic bond.

We begin this book with the epidemiology of shoulder pain and a detailed overview of shoulder anatomy, followed by its biomechanics and motion analysis. Consequently, we delve into clinical problem-solving methods, the use of questionnaires to assess patient outcomes, and the process of screening for potential conditions. The book covers a range of shoulder pathologies, from rotator cuff-related pain and labral injuries to more complex issues like frozen shoulder and glenohumeral instability. With in-depth discussions on diagnostic tools, clinical examinations, and imaging techniques, the book also emphasizes effective communication with patients, highlighting the importance of listening and providing reassurance.

However, it is by no means the intention to be exhaustive. Rare conditions related to the shoulder—such as shoulder pain due to vascular dysfunction—are not discussed or are discussed very briefly. With this book, I aim to provide insight into some of the most common shoulder conditions. Insight that you can then apply to clinically examine your patient with shoulder pain. Insight that you can also convey to your patient, positively influencing the recovery process. Because when the patient understands the problem well, they are much more prone to follow your professional advice. Moreover, this will mean a lot more to the patient because understanding something is the basis for being understood. And it is the foundation for change.

I approach the various shoulder conditions using a consistent and practical method. I address each shoulder condition with the same structure, based on the following questions: what is it, and how can you recognize it in practice?

Contents

About the Author

Filip Struyf, (PhD) is a physical therapist and professor at the Rehabilitation Sciences and Physiotherapy department of the University of Antwerp (Belgium). His profound expertise is the result of years of experience in clinical practice, education, and research. As a passionate researcher, he has dedicated himself to discovering new insights and developing extensive expertise in various shoulder conditions.

He has numerous international and national publications to his name and regularly serves as a speaker at national and international courses and conferences, sharing his knowledge and findings with colleagues. Alongside like-minded professionals, he co-founded the Shoulder Network Flanders, a collaborative effort dedicated to improving shoulder care in Flanders.

Filip Struyf serves as the editor of the book *Frozen Shoulder: Present and Future* and is the author of the in Dutch written book titled *Over de schouder: klinisch onderzoek van een complex gewricht*. This book draws its foundation from the Dutch version of this comprehensive work, showcasing Struyf's expertise in the clinical exploration of the complex aspects of shoulder-related issues. Through his role as both editor and author, Struyf contributes significantly to the understanding and advancement of knowledge in the field of shoulder health and clinical research.

His dedication and expertise have not gone unnoticed. Expertscape, a renowned platform for medical experts, has recognized Filip Struyf as the world's number 1 expert in the field of shoulder pain.

Epidemiology of Shoulder Pain

1

Gaining a profound understanding of the epidemiology of shoulder pain is essential for developing effective prevention and treatment strategies and for improving care and reducing the impact this condition has on individuals and society.

When we refer to shoulder pain, we are not only talking about the specific pain in the shoulder but also its consequences. Patients often experience complaints that go far beyond, such as poor sleep. They wake up when turning on the affected shoulder or struggle to fall asleep due to pain. Sometimes, they withdraw from certain social activities, hobbies, or work. Their daily activities may be affected, including cooking, bathing, dressing, driving, cycling, and more. Additionally, we must not overlook the fact that family members can also "suffer" with the patient, either because they must take on various household tasks or because witnessing their family members suffer affects them emotionally.

But what exactly is shoulder pain? A precise definition of shoulder pain does not exist, and as a result, it is described in many different ways, sometimes based on location, other times on the presumed cause, and perhaps based on the consequences of the complaint. All these variations result in a variety in describing the occurrence of shoulder pain.

The epidemiology of shoulder pain provides insight into the prevalence and incidence of this condition. Shoulder pain is presumed to be the third most common musculoskeletal condition, with an estimated prevalence ranging from 2.5% to 55.2%, depending on the duration of symptoms (average 18%) [2–5]. Only lower back pain and osteoarthritis are more prevalent. Approximately 1–3% of adults consult a general practitioner annually with shoulder pain [3, 4]. So, 1–3% of the adult population on Earth would range between 49 million and 147 million people, every year. And this is an underestimation since not everyone with shoulder pain seeks help. It affects people of all ages and genders, but it occurs slightly more frequently in women and in adults aged 45 and older.

Shoulder pain is also a significant cause of prolonged work absenteeism and disability, resulting in a substantial economic loss. This is not surprising, considering that about 67% of the population will report shoulder complaints at some point in

F. Struyf, *Shoulder Pain*, https://doi.org/10.1007/978-3-031-82228-5_1

their lives, often leading to an inability to work or perform household tasks, thus causing absenteeism, with an estimated annual global financial burden of shoulder pain at around 3 billion dollars [5–8]. In Sweden, the average annual cost per primary care patient (physical therapist or general practitioner) was €4139 (US$4923) based on 2009 tariffs [9]. In the Netherlands, the annual cost of shoulder pain is estimated at €345 million (US$369 million), with absenteeism accounting for around 80% of the total [10]. Inefficiencies in healthcare further add to this economic burden. In Australia, the average annual societal cost for a patient with shoulder pain on waiting lists was AU$7563 (US$4900). For employed patients, this cost increased, ranging from AU$13,885 (US$8995) to AU$22,378 (US$14,500) [11]. However, caution must be applied when translating these figures to other countries due to significant differences in healthcare systems and the wide variation in incurred expenses. The economic cost of shoulder pain can, therefore, vary widely. It is important to note that most epidemiological studies have been conducted in Western Europe, with a few in Asia, Australia, and South America. We lack a significant amount of information from regions such as Africa, Eastern Europe/Russia, and North America.

Furthermore, shoulder pain tends to become chronic in about half of the patients, bringing significant limitations to daily activities and a reduced quality of life. Fortunately, shoulder pain often resolves, and a large portion of patients recover within a few weeks after the onset of symptoms. About half of all patients with shoulder pain achieve full recovery within 6 months of the onset of their complaints, and an additional 10% recover in the following 6 months [10]. However, a significant portion of patients (40%) still experiences persistent pain after 1 year. Some studies have attempted to determine which patients have a longer duration of illness, but prediction models were rarely validated or found useful for clinical practice. One thing is certain: the patient's prognosis depends on more than just structural damage to the shoulder. Consider lifestyle factors, the presence of comorbidities, and psychosocial factors. There is clearly much work to be done in developing validated prognostic prediction models that can take all these different factors into account to identify the most at-risk patients. This could then inform us about tailored advice, approaches, and referrals.

2 Anatomy

In this chapter, we discuss the anatomy of the shoulder in a concise manner, particularly with a focus on what is important for clinical examination. It is by no means the intention to present the complete anatomy of the shoulder. For this purpose, there are other and more comprehensive reference works.

The shoulder joint is the bony link between the upper limb and our trunk. The bone structures that make up the shoulder girdle include the sternum, the clavicle (Fig. 2.1), the scapula (Fig. 2.2), and the humerus (Fig. 2.3).

The following joints are addressed sequentially: the glenohumeral joint, sternoclavicular joint, acromioclavicular joint, and the scapulothoracic gliding surface, along with their associated musculature. The extensive mobility in our shoulder is only achievable when all these bone structures and joints work together. We begin by describing the anatomy of the glenohumeral joint and the labrum.

F. Struyf, *Shoulder Pain*, https://doi.org/10.1007/978-3-031-82228-5_2

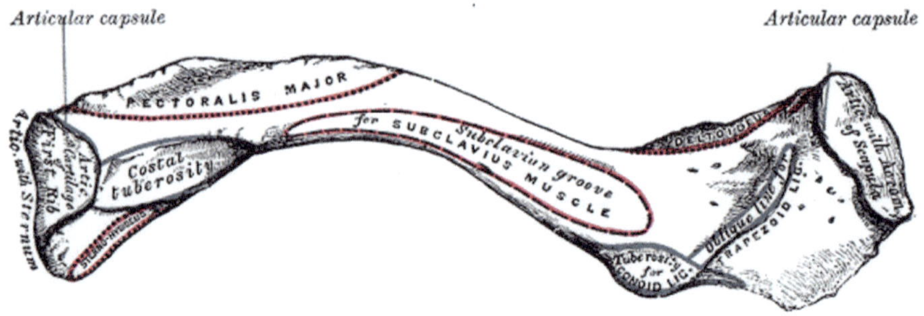

Fig. 2.1 The clavicle

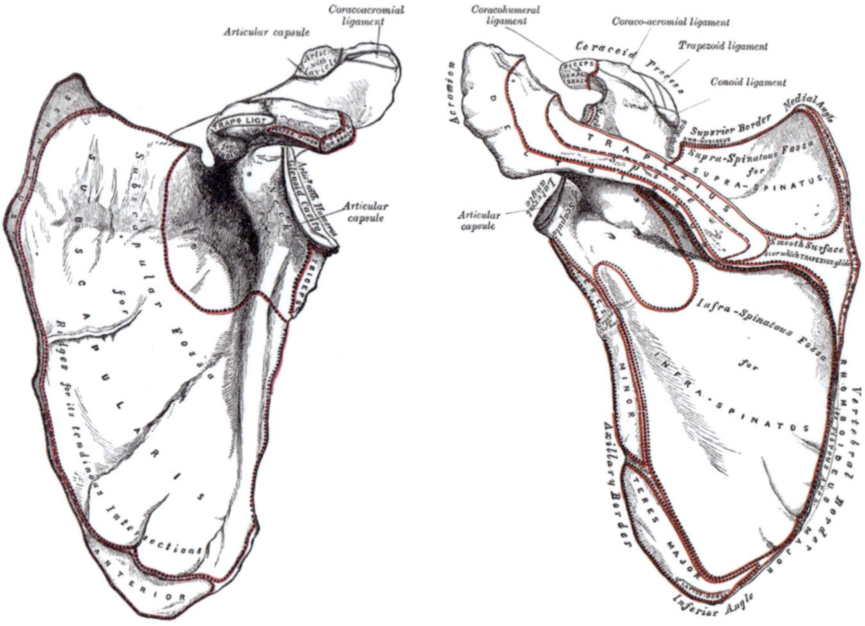

Fig. 2.2 The scapula in front view (right) and rear view (left)

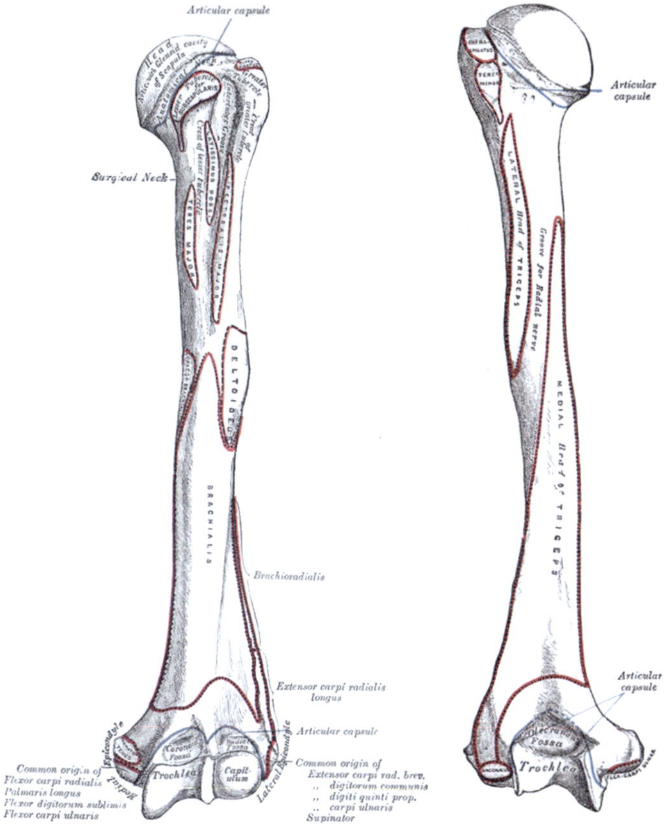

Fig. 2.3 The humerus in frontal view (left) and rear view (right)

The Glenohumeral Joint

The glenohumeral joint is a ball-and-socket joint and consists of the glenoid on the scapula and the humeral head. This joint allows the humerus to move within the glenoid. Both parts have cartilage. The glenoid is much smaller than the humeral head and is oval. The humeral head is three times larger than the glenoid cavity [12]. The diameter is largest in the vertical direction, giving it a somewhat pear-shaped appearance. This contributes to significant mobility, further enhanced by the simultaneous movements of the scapula. To deepen the glenoid and provide a better fit with the humeral head, there is a cartilaginous ring around the glenoid called the labrum. The labrum increases the depth of the glenoid by as much as 50% [13]. The labrum is usually less firmly attached at the upper part and more strongly attached at the lower part of the glenoid. The labrum serves various functions, with three being particularly noteworthy: increasing the contact surface between the humeral head and glenoid, contributing to the “viscoelastic suction effect” (including intra-articular negative pressure), and providing attachment points for stabilizing structures such as the capsule, glenohumeral ligaments, and the long head of the biceps brachii muscle. When an injury occurs, these functions of the labrum are disrupted. Additionally, the labrum serves as an attachment site for various muscles and ligaments. Researchers have even found mechanoreceptors in the labrum, suggesting that the labrum may provide proprioceptive feedback and thus also dynamically contribute to the stability of the glenohumeral joint [14].

The humeral head has a spherical shape and is positioned at an angle of approximately 130 degrees relative to the shaft of the humerus. Additionally, the humeral head is somewhat tilted backward (about 30 degrees) [15]. This largely aligns with the anteriorly oriented glenoid cavity. However, the glenoid cavity is insufficiently concave and too small to be fully congruent with the convex humeral head. Even with the inclusion of an indentation in the socket with elastic cartilage—the glenoid labrum—it is impossible for the entire surface of the humeral head to come into contact with the socket. Sometimes, the analogy of a golf ball on a tee is used. This incongruity of the joint surfaces is additionally compensated for by the joint capsule, ligaments, and muscles.

Surrounding this ball-and-socket joint is a joint capsule (Fig. 2.4), the glenohumeral capsule or "capsula glenohumeralis". This capsule is composed of connective tissue, lined internally with a synovial membrane and filled with synovial fluid. The glenohumeral capsule attaches to the outer edge of the labrum and around the anatomical neck of the humerus while remaining highly flexible. This flexibility is a key factor in the shoulder joint's mobility.

The glenohumeral capsule is reinforced by several ligaments: the coracohumeral ligament (extending from the coracoid process to the greater tubercle of the humerus) (Fig. 2.5), the glenohumeral ligament (consisting of three parts, from the glenoid to the lesser tubercle of the humerus), and the transverse ligament (connecting the greater tubercle to the lesser tubercle, crossing the intertubercular groove, and passing over the long head of the biceps brachii muscle).

The glenohumeral capsule varies in thickness. Generally, it is quite thin (<1 mm), but it does have some thickened areas, such as in the rotator interval. The rotator cable in the rotator interval is described as a crescent-shaped area at the insertion point of the supraspinatus and infraspinatus muscles [16]. This region exhibits a thickening, likely to transfer forces from the supraspinatus and infraspinatus. It is often compared to a suspension bridge that prevents damage to the attachment points, indicating a protective role. It also stabilizes the long head of the biceps brachii tendon.

These thickened portions in the glenohumeral capsule also serve as attachment points for the rotator cuff. However, the ligaments only contribute additional static stability during extreme shoulder movements. The labrum, ligaments, and glenohumeral capsule are often collectively referred to as the static stabilizers of the glenohumeral joint. Nonetheless, it should not be overlooked that, like the labrum, mechanoreceptors have been found in the capsule and ligaments, suggesting that they also play a role in dynamic stability.

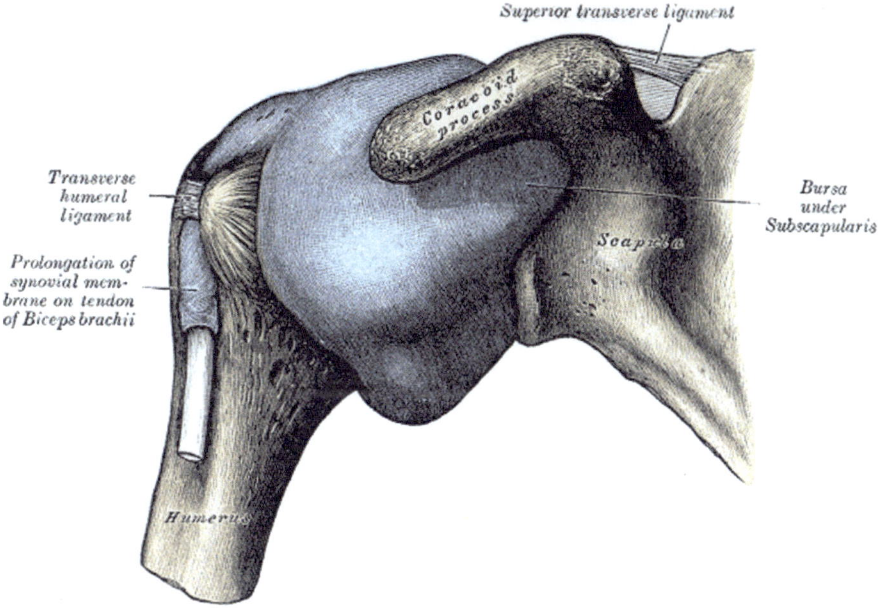

Fig. 2.4 The glenohumeral joint in frontal view

Fig. 2.5 The cavitas glenoidalis in lateral view

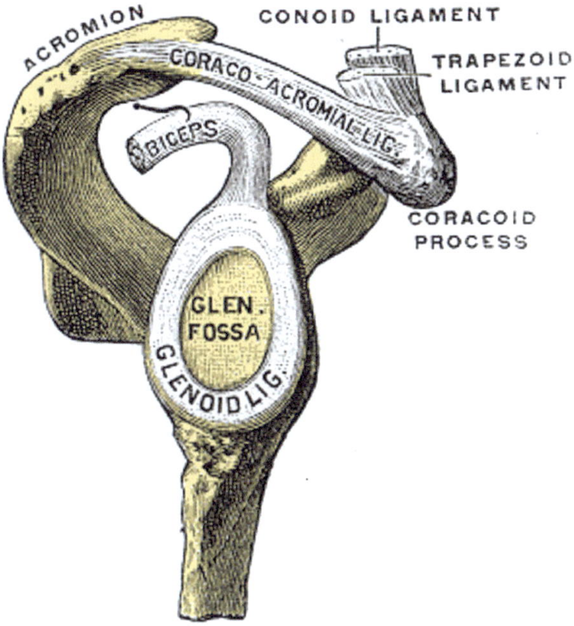

The significance of this region is increasingly highlighted in the literature due to the relationship between injuries to the rotator cable and patient complaints. The extent of this relationship, however, is not yet strongly proven. There is suspicion that rotator cuff tears affecting the rotator cable also have an increased risk of recurrence after recovery. The integrity of the rotator cable is also linked to the phenomenon of pseudoparalysis, where patients have limited active mobility. Dynamic stability, on the other hand, is provided by a series of muscles, notably the rotator cuff. The rotator cuff consists of four muscles: the supraspinatus muscle, infraspinatus muscle, teres minor muscle, and subscapularis muscle. These muscles originate laterally on the humeral head and converge with the fibrous glenohumeral joint capsule, as well as with each other [17]. Posteriorly, the supraspinatus, infraspinatus, and teres minor muscles unite just before their attachment to the greater tubercle of the humerus. Anteriorly, the supraspinatus and subscapularis muscles also form a sheath that surrounds the long head of the biceps brachii muscle in the bicipital groove [18].

Additionally, the glenohumeral joint is enveloped by the deltoid muscle, a large superficial muscle with fibers on the front, back, and at the side of the shoulder. It originates from the lower part of the spine of the scapula, acromion, and lateral part of the clavicle, running to the deltoid tuberosity on the humerus. This allows the deltoid muscle to abduct, internally rotate, externally rotate the arm, and perform ante—and retroflexion with a significant lever. In addition, the long head of the biceps brachii (from the supraglenoid tubercle to the radius) and short head of the biceps brachii (from the coracoid process to the radius) (Fig. 2.6), the triceps brachii muscle (from the infraglenoid tubercle and posterior side of the humerus to the ulna) (Fig. 2.7), and the coracobrachialis muscle (from the coracoid process to the middle/medial side of the humerus) play a significant role in shoulder flexion and extension.

The long head of the biceps brachii muscle makes a considerable twist from its muscular belly to its attachment, especially with the arm in a neutral position. This region is often the site of tendinopathies affecting the long head of the biceps brachii muscle. Finally, the humerus is controlled by three internal rotators/adductors: the pectoralis major muscle (from the clavicle, sternocostal region, and sternum to the crest of the tubercle), latissimus dorsi muscle (Fig. 2.8) (from the transverse processes of T7–T12, thoracolumbar fascia, and iliac crest, ribs 10–12 to the crest of the lesser tubercle on the humerus), and the teres major muscle (from laterally on the inferior angle of the scapula to the crest of the lesser tubercle).

Ruptures of the pectoralis major muscle are relatively rare injuries but are increasingly reported in young male patients after experiencing high loads on the muscle, particularly during weightlifting or bench pressing [19].

The glenohumeral joint also features a series of bursae, with the subacromial-deltoid bursa being the most well-known among them. Bursae facilitate movements in areas where there might otherwise be considerable friction. Thus, we identify the subacromial-deltoid bursa, subscapular bursa, coracobrachial bursa, and, finally, the subcoracoid bursa. Little is known about most bursae, except for the subacromial-deltoid bursa. The upper boundary of this bursa is delineated by the acromion, the

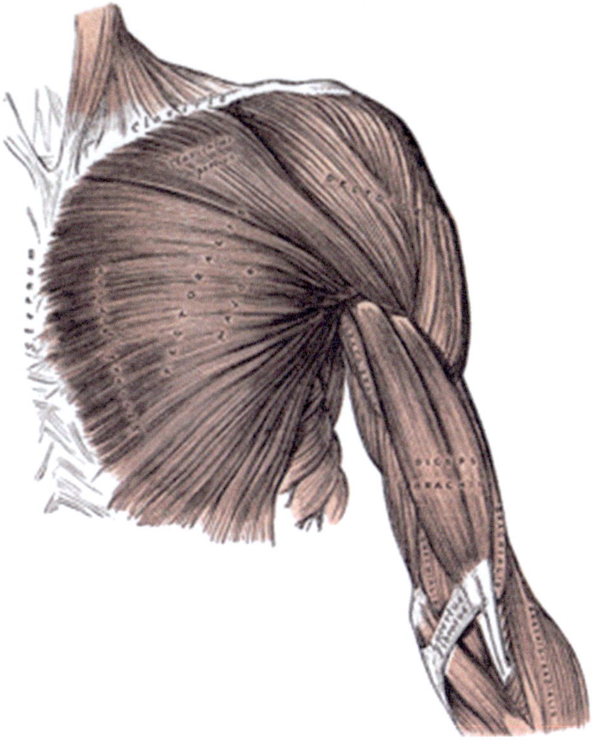

Fig. 2.6 The pectoralis major muscle, biceps brachii muscle, and deltoid muscle

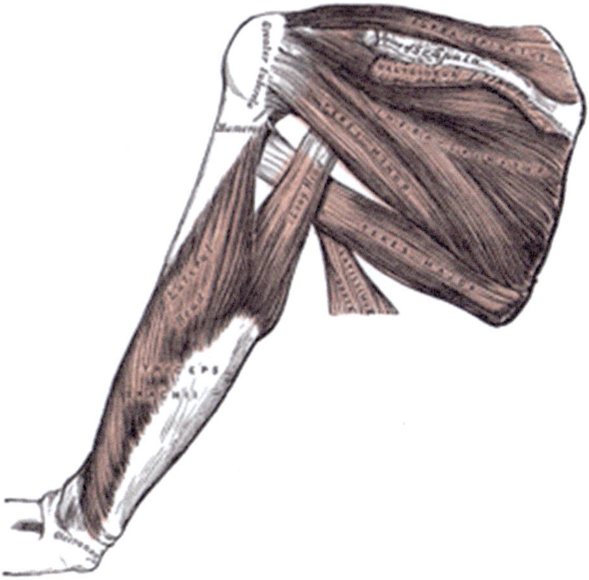

Fig. 2.7 Triceps brachii muscle, supraspinatus muscle, infraspinatus muscle, teres minor muscle, and teres major muscle

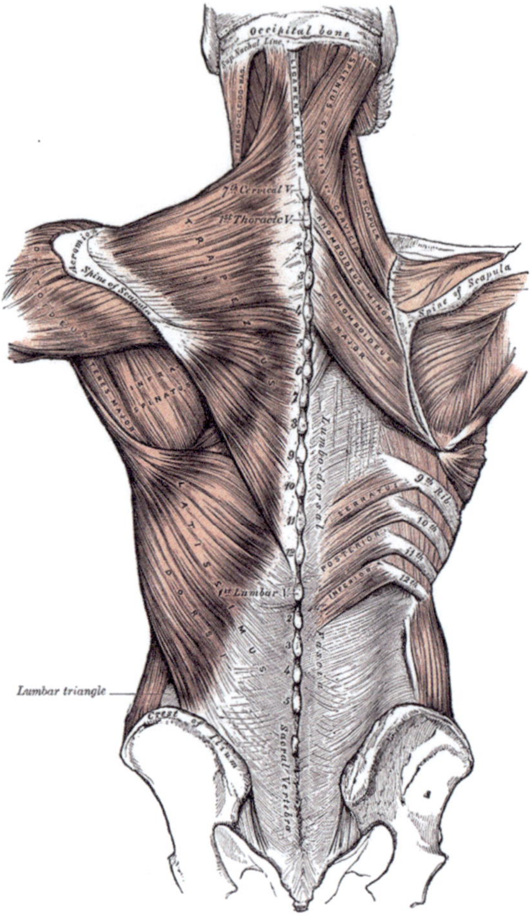

Fig. 2.8 The trapezius muscle, latissimus dorsi muscle, rhomboid muscles, and levator scapulae muscle

coracoid process, and the coracoacromial ligament in between. At the lower boundary, the rotator cuff rests against the humeral head. The bursa itself is lined on the inside with a synovial membrane. The upper layer of the bursa thus runs together with the lower epimysium of the deltoid muscle, while the lower layer runs with that of the rotator cuff. Due to a thin layer with synovial fluid, there is optimal sliding between both muscular structures.

The Acromioclavicular and Sternoclavicular Joints

The acromioclavicular joint (AC joint) (Fig. 2.9) is the joint between the acromion and the clavicle. Both ends are covered with cartilage. In some individuals, a fibrocartilaginous disc is found, while in others, the disc may be incomplete, smaller, or

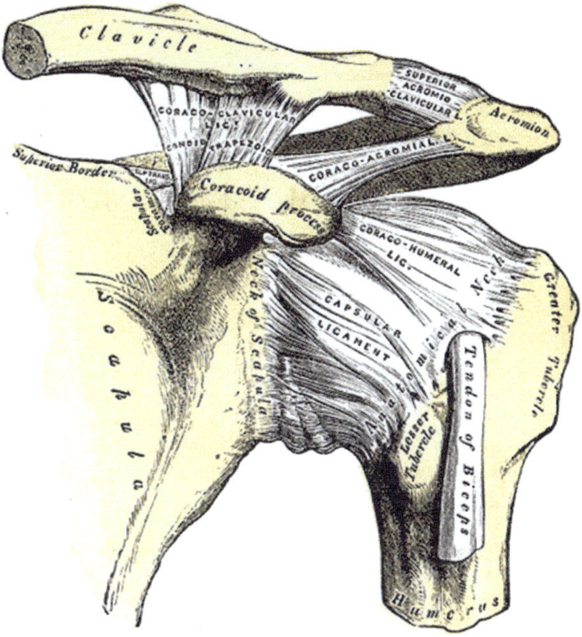

Fig. 2.9 The acromioclavicular joint and the ligamentous structures around the glenohumeral joint

even absent altogether. The disc between the ends enhances congruence. Surrounding the AC joint, there is a robust joint capsule and a series of ligaments that further strengthen it: the acromiocoracoid ligament, acromioclavicular ligament, and coracoclavicular ligament (conoid and trapezoid ligaments). This joint connects the scapula (and consequently the entire arm) to the thorax.

The sternoclavicular joint (SC joint) (Fig. 2.10) is the joint between the sternum and the clavicle, reinforced by two ligaments: the anterior and posterior sternoclavicular ligament and a fibrocartilaginous disc. It is a saddle joint in terms of shape but could also be seen as a ball-and-socket joint due to the range of motion it permits in multiple directions.

The Scapulothoracic Joint

The scapulothoracic joint is not a synovial joint but rather a physiological joint that consists of the scapula and the thorax. The scapula is a large bone that serves as both the attachment site for various scapulothoracic and glenohumeral muscles and positions the glenoid to allow the humerus to move with sufficient congruence. The scapulothoracic muscles include the trapezius muscle (from the occiput, nuchal ligament, and the spinous processes of C7–T12 to the upper part of the spine of the scapula, acromion, and lateral part of the clavicle), rhomboid muscles (major and

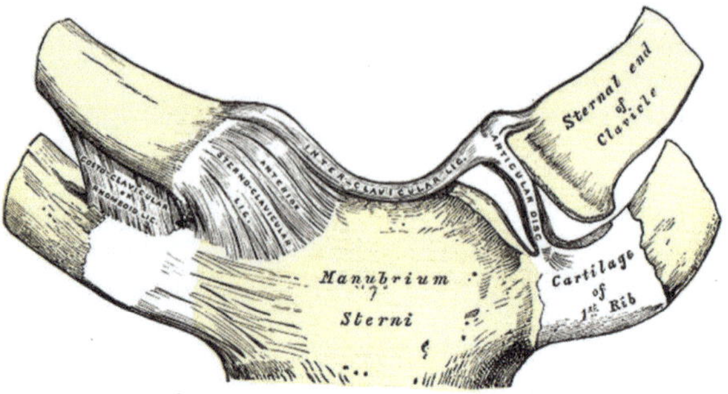

Fig. 2.10 The sternoclavicular joints

minor; from spinous processes of C6–T4 to the medial border of the scapula), pectoralis minor muscle (from the costosternal junction of ribs 3–5 to the coracoid process), levator scapulae muscle (from transverse processes of C1–C4 to the superior angle of the scapula), and serratus anterior muscle (from ribs 1–9 to the inner medial border of the scapula).

Neuroanatomy of the Shoulder Region

While most shoulder conditions are not directly related to nerve disorders, it is still important to have knowledge of the various nerves that pass through our shoulder and may give rise to a neurogenic pain pattern.

The innervation of the upper limb originates primarily from our cervical region. Large nerve trunks, specifically the brachial plexus (Fig. 2.11), arise from C3 to Th1, consisting of upper, middle, and lower trunks. Supraclavicular, various branches form, such as the dorsal scapular nerve and the suprascapular nerve. Below the clavicle, we describe a posterior, lateral, and medial bundle, leading to further branching. Approximately at the level of our axillary fold, these bundles divide into the median nerve, radial nerve, axillary nerve, ulnar nerve, and musculocutaneous nerve. Below is an overview of the main neurological structures around the shoulder. The ulnar nerve and median nerve only innervate muscles in the forearm and will not be further discussed here.

The accessory nerve (n. accessorius) has both sensory and motor functions, innervating the trapezius muscle and sternocleidomastoid muscle. Clinical manifestation of its dysfunction includes head tilt and difficulty raising the arm above 90 degrees due to a lack of scapular upward rotation.

The dorsal scapular nerve (n. dorsalis scapulae) innervates the rhomboideus major, rhomboideus minor, and levator scapulae muscles. Damage to the dorsal scapular nerve may result in scapular dyskinesia and limited movement due to a lack of scapular contribution to overall shoulder movement.

The long thoracic nerve (n. thoracicus longus) innervates the serratus anterior muscle. The serratus anterior muscle primarily functions to stabilize the scapula against the thorax but also to upwardly rotate the scapula. Injury, such as a fall on

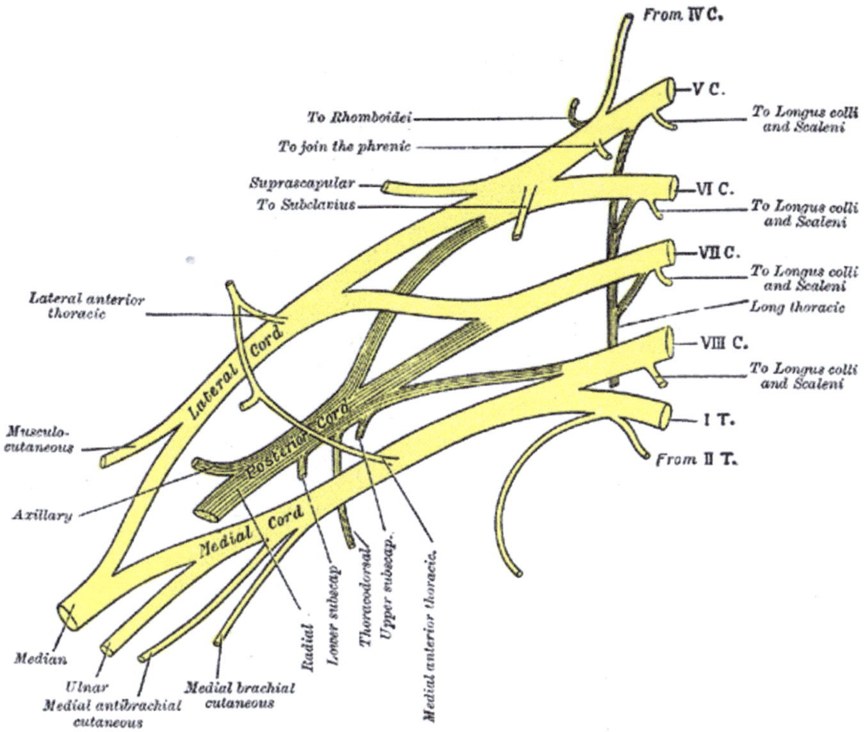

Fig. 2.11 Overview of the brachial plexus

the ribs with an extended arm, can lead to noticeable scapular winging, where the medial border of the scapula moves away from the thorax toward internal scapular rotation. Prolonged heavy lifting or surgical procedures are other potential causes of damage to the long thoracic nerve, resulting in inflammation and weakness of the serratus anterior muscle, potentially involving the deltoid muscle, biceps brachii, and part of the rotator cuff. Pain or numbness may also occur.

The axillary nerve (n. axillaris) innervates the deltoid muscle and teres minor muscle. It also provides sensory function around the inferior part of the deltoid muscle. Axillary nerve damage can occur, for example, following nerve injury from trauma, such as a fall on an outstretched arm while protecting the head.

The radial nerve (n. radialis) innervates the triceps brachii, brachialis, brachioradialis, and various extensor muscles of the forearm. It provides sensory innervation to the back of the forearm and hand (excluding the pinky side). Radial nerve injury can be caused in various ways. Injury at the axillary fold is sometimes referred to as Saturday night palsy, resulting from prolonged pressure in the armpit, as seen in deep sleep after alcohol consumption. Patients may experience weakness in elbow and wrist extension. Sensory loss may be evident on the lateral back of the forearm and hand (excluding the pinky side).

The musculocutaneous nerve (n. musculocutaneus) innervates the coracobrachialis, biceps brachii, and part of the brachialis. It provides sensation to the lateral side of the forearm. Overloading (trauma or microtrauma) of these muscles can lead to irritation or damage to this nerve, causing pain or tingling around the lateral forearm. Complaints may worsen with elbow flexion, not to be confused with a tendinopathic condition.

The suprascapular nerve (n. suprascapularis) innervates the supraspinatus and infraspinatus muscles. Clinical damage or impingement may lead to weakness and atrophy of these muscles, accompanied by pain on the dorsal side.

The subscapular nerve (n. subscapularis) innervates the latissimus dorsi (thoracodorsal nerve), subscapularis, and teres major muscles.

The pectoral nerves (nn. pectorales) innervate the pectoralis major and minor muscles. These nerves are usually divided into lateral and medial branches. The lateral branch innervates the pectoralis major, while the medial branch innervates the pectoralis minor. Damage can occur during surgery or trauma.

3 Motion Analysis

In this chapter, we briefly address the motion analysis of the shoulder, focusing on what is essential for clinical examination. Building upon the anatomy, we discuss the glenohumeral joint, sternoclavicular joint, acromioclavicular joint, and the scapulothoracic articulation.

As a general rule, more mobility often comes at the expense of stability. This is a characteristic phenomenon when observing the shoulder. The shoulder exhibits remarkable mobility, but it is evident that this comes at the cost of structural stability in the joint.

The Glenohumeral Joint

The glenohumeral joint is a ball-and-socket joint. This means that the humeral head moves like a ball in the glenoid cavity. When you abduct your arm, the ball will roll upward in the cavity. If it only rolls without proper control, it can dislocate. To prevent this, the humeral head makes a downward sliding movement to stay securely in the socket. In addition to the typically described rotations, translations are also observable in the glenohumeral joint. Proper functioning of the shoulder is only possible when the head stays within the socket. When lowering the arm, the reverse occurs: the humeral head rolls downward and slides upward. This upward sliding is often referred to as translation.

We just described superior and inferior translations, but during movements like internal and external rotation, as well as anteflexion and retroflexion, anterior and posterior translations are also necessary. During an anteflexion movement, the anterior fibers of the deltoid muscle pull the humeral head forward, and then the posterior cuff keeps the humeral head in place with a posteriorly oriented translational movement.

F. Struyf, *Shoulder Pain*, https://doi.org/10.1007/978-3-031-82228-5_3

The Sternoclavicular and Acromioclavicular Joints

The sternoclavicular and acromioclavicular (AC) joints are smaller joints but are no less important for the proper functioning of the shoulder. Generally, the scapula is connected with the sternum via the clavicle. When we abduct the arm, our clavicle will move a few degrees upward (approximately 13 degrees), tilt posteriorly (approximately 20 degrees), and rotate posteriorly around its axis (approximately 20 degrees) [20]. Our clavicle makes a unique movement in the joint with our sternum. This is a saddle joint. This means that the clavicle, as it moves upward, rolls superiorly and slides inferiorly, but when it tilts posteriorly, it simultaneously rolls and slides posteriorly. Imagine a horse rider on your clavicle looking toward your neck. When that rider tilts forward, they will roll forward in the saddle but slide backward to stay in the saddle. However, sideways does not involve the same inverse movement: the rider will slide/roll sideways without a counteracting motion.

At the AC joint, our clavicle lies on the acromion. Basically, the clavicle follows the movements of the scapula. The movements of the clavicle are essential for a well-functioning scapulothoracic joint and, consequently, the entire shoulder. The clavicle is, after all, the only bony contact between the shoulder and our torso. The clavicle articulates with the acromion of our scapula, thus supporting the movements of the scapula. As much as one-third of our total shoulder mobility is attributed to our acromioclavicular and sternoclavicular joints [21].

The Scapulothoracic Joint

The position of our scapula is mainly determined by the shape of our thorax, the muscle action around our scapula, and the AC joint. This positioning is crucial to centralize the humeral head and create a stable base for various shoulder movements [22]. There is no ideal resting position of the scapula and no ideal scapulothoracic movement. Indeed, there is a significant variety that falls within the limits of normal.

Scapular movements are always described in relation to the thorax. During the upward movement of our arm, the scapula undergoes upward rotation (the cavity points upward). During the descent of our arm, the scapula undergoes downward rotation (the cavity points downward). Furthermore, during the upward lift, the scapula also tilts backward (posterior tilting), and, conversely, it tilts forward (anterior tilting). Finally, the scapula also rotates around its axis inward and outward, but these movements often depend on the direction in which we move our arm. An anteflexion movement will mainly be characterized by scapular internal rotation, while an abduction movement will mostly involve scapular external rotation. We cannot rotate our scapula upward or downward without moving our humerus. This once again demonstrates the strong functional interdependence between the scapula and the glenohumeral joint.

The position and movements of the scapula often differ between individuals with and without shoulder pain [23]. This is often a consequence of shoulder pain, but it can just as well be the cause of the complaints. Moreover, there can be altered scapular movement even when someone does not have shoulder pain. Even the speed of your movement can make the scapula rotate differently. You can compare it to our way of walking. Everyone walks a bit differently, and that does not necessarily lead to complaints. But if you have a lot of pain somewhere, you may start to limp. And as you start walking faster or get tired, your hips, knees, and feet will also make different angles. In some conditions, these altered scapular movements are particularly evident, such as in patients with restricted glenohumeral mobility (as in a frozen shoulder), where they compensate by clearly making faster use of their scapulothoracic mobility.

Muscle Functioning Around the Shoulder

Our shoulder consists of an extensive number of muscles and twice as many tendons. Whether a muscle contributes to a shoulder movement depends on the direction of the movement, the position of the arm, and the force moment of the respective muscle. The rotator cuff muscles and tendons are the most frequently affected. They owe their name to their presumed function: rotation in the shoulder. Although they play a role in this function, this nomenclature can be misleading regarding their actual function: keeping the humeral head in the socket during various arm movements.

Firstly, there is a large and powerful deltoid muscle . This muscle primarily allows us to move our shoulder outward, forward, or backward, thanks to the many muscle fibers at the front and back of our shoulder. Additionally, we have the large pectoral muscle, the pectoralis major, which primarily adducts and internally rotates our arm. At the back, we have the very large latissimus dorsi muscle, a muscle that can also internally rotate our arm and perform retroflexion. We use the latissimus dorsi extensively when pulling ourselves up physically.

In a muscle layer beneath the deltoid, our rotator cuff emerges. As you have read, its main goal is to keep the humeral head in its socket. But why is this so crucial? Well, the large muscles we mentioned earlier, which attach to the upper arm, have a significant lever effect. This means that when these large and strong muscles contract, they can, in a way, pull our humeral head out of its socket. If this were to happen, the shoulder would dislocate, rendering it practically immobile. To prevent this, in addition to the aforementioned static stabilizers, we have our rotator cuff. A well-functioning rotator cuff must be strong enough to keep the humeral head in its socket. However, strength alone is not enough. They must contract at the right moment and collaborate effectively. They are team players. During abduction, a well-functioning rotator cuff prevents the deltoid from moving the humerus superiorly. The rotator cuff also keeps the humerus centered medially in the socket.

You can compare it to a puppet on a string. The hand above is our large strong muscles (deltoid, pectoralis major, latissimus dorsi), and the fingers/strings are our rotator cuff. When the hand does nothing, the fingers should do no more than carry the puppet. When the hand moves left and right or up and down, the fingers must act to keep the puppet stable. This is how our rotator cuff works. The more powerful our large muscles contract, the more powerful the rotator cuff must work. We will delve deeper into the rotator cuff in the chapter on its tendon problems.

We must not overlook two equally important muscles as the rotator cuff: the biceps brachii and the triceps brachii. Firstly, they have a function at the elbow level: the biceps brachii flexes the elbow and supinates our forearm; the triceps brachii extends the elbow. Then, these muscles also have a function at shoulder level. The biceps brachii will contribute to shoulder anteflexion, and the triceps brachii, on the other hand, contributes to retroflexion of the upper arm. However, due to the intra-articular course of the long head of the biceps brachii, it will have limited leverage and, therefore, limited impact on these movements. The biceps' action will also depend on the elbow position. When the elbow is in flexion and supination, the biceps brachii will have a limited ability to exert force and stabilize the glenohumeral joint.

In summary, it is suspected that both muscles have a role in stabilizing the humeral head in its socket. Especially the long head of the biceps brachii would assist in stabilizing the humeral head [24]. According to some researchers, this function becomes significant when we have already raised our arm almost to shoulder height, such as during overhead movements. The tendon will then change from a curvilinear course to a straighter course.

Finally, we have our scapulothoracic muscles. These play a crucial role in the movements and position of the shoulder blade. The trapezius, together with the serratus anterior, forms a force couple that upwardly rotates the scapula and dynamically fixes it against the thorax. So, it is primarily these muscles that help guide the humeral head within the cavity and provides stability. It involves a collaboration of different scapulothoracic muscles, where no single muscle could perform the task on its own. Since the rotator cuff originates from the scapula, the scapulothoracic muscles also ensure that the rotator cuff always has an efficient length-tension relationship. Only in this way can the rotator cuff work efficiently and effectively, by keeping the humeral head nicely in its socket.

From the paragraphs above, it might almost seem that all strength, control, and mobility are attributed to the shoulder itself. However, there is ample evidence that the shoulder is part of a larger musculoskeletal system and, therefore, does not work in isolation. For example, half of the force generated by the upper limb during a tennis serve comes from the lower limbs and trunk [25]. And there is increasing evidence that shoulder complaints may originate elsewhere in the body [26–30]. The idea here stems from the energy flow from the lower limbs to the hands. Overhead athletes with injuries to the lower limbs indeed seem to have a higher risk of shoulder complaints [31]. Therefore, when evaluating a patient with shoulder pain, we must not overlook the impact of the entire musculoskeletal system, the so-called kinetic chain.

4 Problem-Solving

The clinician examines and analyzes the patient's movement and functioning possibilities, focusing on the causes of health problems and their consequences. In order to arrive at the most likely hypothesis, they approach it consciously, procedurally, systematically, and targeted.

A targeted approach implies that the healthcare provider knows the goal they want to achieve. They guide their actions based on a concrete idea of the result to be achieved with their intervention. Preferably, they discuss this with the patient.

Consciousness indicates that the healthcare provider is aware of what is going on within themselves, their own values, and their norms. They are also aware of the patient, their situation, and the potential consequences of their actions. It is important for the clinician to be aware that their actions can lead to unintended but desired effects, or intended and desired, as well as unintended and undesired effects.

Systematic means that the healthcare provider acts according to a logical sequence of steps related to the goals. They use certain rules or methods, relying on a coherent set of beliefs and principles. This allows the healthcare provider to avoid unnecessary interventions.

Finally, a procedural approach means that the healthcare provider understands the developments over time and bases their actions on them. This implies that outcomes and data from the previous phase of the examination have implications for the future course of the investigation. Also, in the case of interventions, the clinician acts procedurally, enabling them to make an assessment for the next intervention based on the results of the previous one.

Patients typically come to us with a problem that needs resolution. Various strategies exist for problem-solving. Using a strategy means that, based on prevailing circumstances, a specific plan and approach are followed to achieve a goal. First and foremost, it must be clear what the problem is. It must be recognized and formulated. A distinction is made between the problem the patient presents—their health problem—and the problem the clinician faces: determining the patient's health problem, understanding its structure, and how to resolve it. Possible strategies to

F. Struyf, *Shoulder Pain*, https://doi.org/10.1007/978-3-031-82228-5_4

solve a problem include the hypothetico-deductive approach, pattern recognition, the algorithm or decision tree, and the gathering method.

The Hypothetico-Deductive Approach

In the hypothetico-deductive approach, you formulate hypotheses right from the beginning regarding what the problem is and which aspects are interconnected and play a role in the problem. You also develop hypotheses about solutions to the problem. A hypothesis is an explicit assumption. Subsequently, the hypothesis is further delineated and adjusted through deduction. The hypothetico-deductive method is suggested to be an effective way to solve the patient's problem.

In healthcare, complex problems are the standard. To address these problems, it must be clear what problem or problems are at hand (presenting problem). The problem is defined, and in the case of multiple issues, priorities are established. For problem analysis, various alternative hypotheses are initiatlly formulated, leaving multiple options open. Subsequently, efforts are made to investigate precisely those aspects that narrow down the options and establish the most probable hypothesis. A drawback of this method is its dependence on knowledge about the hypotheses. A healthcare provider with limited knowledge about hypotheses may formulate restricted or erroneous hypotheses.

Pattern Recognition

Pattern recognition refers to recognizing a problem based on previous experiences. There is an immediate realization that the symptoms and presentation of the patient match those of a similar problem. Especially experienced clinicians utilize pattern recognition to solve the patient's problem. Conscious pattern recognition of problems, causes, and solutions, learned through theoretical knowledge and reinforced by clinical experience, can be a characteristic of expert clinical practice. However, the danger of this approach is that only those symptoms that fit the assumed familiar problem are recognized, and symptoms contradicting it may be overlooked. This risk is relatively high not only for less experienced clinicians but also for more experienced colleagues, particularly after attending a specific course on a particular condition. After such a course, the clinician is more likely to interpret the patient's complaints as fitting the pattern associated with the recently learned condition.

The Algorithm

An algorithm or decision tree strategy refers to the clinician arriving at the correct conclusion or diagnosis by following a diagnostic process. In this case, the different paths are predefined: decision tree, flowchart, or algorithm. The decision tree consists of an initial question, followed by steps such as if no, then proceed to step x, if yes, then proceed to step y. For this, the steps and their various consequences must be clear and unambiguous. Algorithms are increasingly being developed in healthcare. Algorithms are an excellent way to visually represent the structure of a specific condition. Some symptoms of a particular condition are less likely to be overlooked using algorithms. However, there are significant limitations to this problem-solving method. Algorithms are particularly useful in the case of a limited number of variables, as in this traffic example: green light means go, red light means stop, and orange light means the algorithm splits here depending on the distance and speed at which you are driving. However, some additional variables need to be considered, such as the presence of a tram, bus, or ambulance. It becomes clear that the algorithm becomes complicated and challenging to work with, especially with about a dozen variables. The complexity of a patient seeking help involves hundreds, perhaps even thousands of variables. Therefore, it is logical that an algorithm provides a view of the actual situation that is too simplistic.

The Gathering Method

Finally, with the gathering method, the complete medical history and the current state of functioning are examined (without immediately focusing on outcomes), ultimately leading to a diagnosis. This reduces the likelihood of overlooking something. Only when all information is obtained can a conclusion be formulated. However, it is an unguided method, leading to inefficient and ineffective actions, unnecessarily burdening patients. Such an approach is generally not recommended.

> In summary, clinicians should strive to recognize clinical patterns (as presented in this book) but should be cautious about relying solely on them. A so-called tunnel vision can make it difficult to recognize new patterns. Therefore, we recommend maintaining a balance between pattern recognition and the hypothetico-deductive approach.

5 Questionnaires, PROMS, and PREMS

When a patient completes a questionnaire, you obtain a result, an outcome. This outcome serves as an indicator to assess changes in health status or quality of life. Questionnaires are often used in intervention studies or longitudinal studies, but they could also be an integral part of routine clinical care.

In the past, questionnaires mainly focused on biomedical factors. Nowadays, most outcomes for individuals with chronic conditions consist of questionnaires measuring multiple aspects of the consequences of the condition. In this book, a questionnaire is defined as a *patient-reported outcome measure* (PROM), which consolidates a series of items into a total score, subscores, or both.

When suspecting a shoulder problem, various questionnaires can be employed to obtain a standardized overview of the patient's complaints. Indeed, it is advisable to have the patient complete such a questionnaire. The results not only provide answers to questions that may have been overlooked during the medical history but also offer a general idea of the patient's complaints (based on the total score of the questionnaire). This general idea can then be used to estimate progress by administering the same questionnaire at different time points. To monitor and assess a patient's shoulder condition, clinicians can use various reliable and valid PROMs for shoulder injuries. However, their validity is also related to the language in which they are provided and studied, as well as by the characteristics of the patient population. This means that a questionnaire validated in English may not be validated in another language or vice versa. In this book, we focus on questionnaires that are reliable and valid in English and are relevant to patients with a specific shoulder condition.

Similar to a clinical test, a questionnaire should be used with caution. In addition to a specific range and reliability, a questionnaire also has a *standard error of measurement* (SEM), *minimal detectable change* (MDC), and *minimal clinically important difference* (MCID). Without an understanding of these concepts and their respective values, clinical decision-making can go wrong. These concepts are summarized below.

Whenever a patient completes a questionnaire, there is a chance of a measurement error, the SEM. The SEM of a questionnaire is a statistical measure indicating

F. Struyf, *Shoulder Pain*, https://doi.org/10.1007/978-3-031-82228-5_5

the average amount of error that typically occurs when filling out a questionnaire. The higher the SEM of a questionnaire, the less accurate it is. Since the SEM depends on the variance of scores obtained from repeated measurements, the SEM is calculated based on reliability (ICC) and standard deviation (SD) in the respective population. This shows how the patient's score may fluctuate above or below the true value.

Standard error of measurement = SEM = $(\mathrm{SD} \times \sqrt{1} - \mathrm{ICC})$.

Subsequently, the SEM allows you to calculate the minimal detectable change, the MDC. The MDC refers to the smallest change in a measuring instrument that can be reliably detected and is not due to the SEM. The MDC represents the threshold of change that must be exceeded to be confident that the detected change is not due to measurement error. Usually, the MDC is supplemented with the confidence interval, for example, MDC90. This means you are 90% confident that the correct score of the questionnaire will lie within this interval.

Minimal detectable difference = MDC90 = $(1.64 \times \mathrm{SEM} \times \sqrt{2})$

The MCID, on the other hand, refers to the smallest change in the score of a questionnaire considered meaningful to the patient. The MCID is determined through analyses of patient populations. In other words, the MCID objectifies at what change in the score on a PROM the patient actually feels better.

The difference between measurement 1 and measurement 2 must be greater than the MDC and MCID to avoid being the result of a systematic error and to be clinically relevant, respectively. It is important to note that reported values of SEM, MDC, and MCID may vary between different studies as they depend on the population under investigation.

An example:

A patient with a frozen shoulder completes the Shoulder Pain and Disability Index (SPADI) and scores 60/100. The MDC90 is 18.1 [32]. The MCID ranges between 14 and 21/100 [33]. The MDC90 informs us with 90% certainty that the true score lies between 41.9 and 78.1/100. When the patient notes a score of 40/100 after a few weeks, we know that this is not due to measurement error but represents a genuine improvement. Moreover, the improvement exceeds the MCID. This allows us to conclude that the improvement is not due to a systematic error and is also clinically relevant. The patient is likely to perceive it as a real and meaningful improvement.

In addition to well-known PROMs, there is an increasing use of patient-reported experience measures (PREMs). PROMs focus on assessing symptoms, functions, and health-related quality of life, while PREMs capture the patient's perspective on how the care has been provided and evaluate the effect of care delivery [34]. Facilitating such communication channels promotes patient-centered care. For example, living with shoulder pain can have profound psychological consequences, including feelings of frustration, anxiety, reduced self-esteem, irritability, and depression. Consider patients with a frozen shoulder, where persistent pain and interrupted sleep can influence the patient's mood. Qualitative studies suggest that patients with a frozen shoulder often feel that the severity of their symptoms is not understood. They frequently experience a lack of empathy and understanding from family, friends, colleagues, and healthcare providers [35]. Health workers also often tend to downplay the severity of symptoms and fail to acknowledge their impact. This can contribute to a negative self-image and feelings of hopelessness in the patient, which are counterproductive to the therapeutic relationship. Understanding the patient's experience is crucial for effective treatment. If a patient feels that their struggle is understood, it can have profound positive consequences [36]. In this context, PREMS can be particularly useful, as they help capture the patient's perspective on their care, making it easier for healthcare providers to address concerns and build a stronger, more empathetic therapeutic relationship.

Questionnaires Focusing on (Shoulder) Pain

Visual Analog Scale

A scoring system that is useful for every shoulder condition is the visual analog scale (VAS) (Fig. 5.1). Shoulder pain is measured on a 100 mm VAS, ranging from 0 (no pain) to 100 (the worst imaginable pain). Since this method has been used and studied in a wide range of populations, the MDC and MCID can vary depending on the studied population. On average, the MCID for the VAS is estimated to be 14 mm in patients with rotator cuff complaints [37].

Numeric Pain Rating Scale

The Numerical Pain Rating Scale (NPRS) is a patient-reported outcome measure (PROM) with scores ranging from 1 to 10. Unlike the VAS, the NPRS can be administered verbally. Usually, a 7-day timeframe is used, with a question like "How would you rate your pain on average over the last 7 days?"

The same extremes apply as with the VAS: from no pain to the worst imaginable pain. This scoring method is easy to handle during history taking and has proven to be reliable, valid, and responsive in patients with shoulder pain [38]. The MDC90 and MCID are 2 and 1 point, respectively. The difference between two measurements must be greater than 2 to avoid being attributed to measurement error and to be clinically relevant.

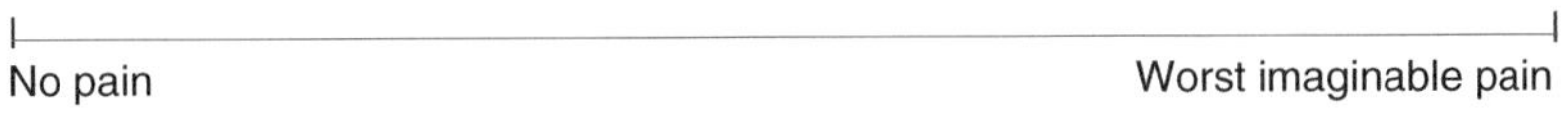

Fig. 5.1 Visual analog scale (100 mm)

Brief Pain Inventory

The Brief Pain Inventory (BPI) aims to assess pain intensity and the impact of pain on daily life (quality of life). The BPI is mainly tested in chronic pain populations, such as fibromyalgia or osteoarthritis, but also in postoperative painful conditions. The BPI is reliable, valid, and responsive, with a MCID of 2.2 in patients with MSK disorders [39].

Combined Scoring Systems

Constant-Murley Score

The Constant-Murley Score, or simply the Constant Score, is perhaps the most popular questionnaire that evaluates the functioning of patients with shoulder pain. It consists of two parts: one completed by the patient (35 points) and another part filled out by the healthcare provider based on clinical testing (65 points). The higher the score, the better the shoulder function.

Unfortunately, popularity does not guarantee quality. Many variations in measurement methods have been described, and the lack of standardized use has led to much criticism of this scoring method [40]. Additionally, there are also no published data on its ability to detect change (e.g., MDC or MCID). If you decide to use this scoring method, it is essential to ensure proper standardization of the second part.

Questionnaires Focusing on Functioning of the Shoulder or Upper Limb

Shoulder Pain and Disability Index

The Shoulder Pain and Disability Index (SPADI) assesses the presence of pain intensity and shoulder function. This instrument is a standardized questionnaire consisting of 13 items, with each item scored from 0 to 10. The SPADI is divided in two subdomains: a pain scale and a function scale. The composite SPADI score ranges from 0 to 100, where higher scores indicate greater pain and reduced functioning. The ability of the SPADI to detect change varies considerably depending on the study [41]. The minimal detectable change at 95% confidence level (MDC95) ranges from 13.2 to 21.5 [41]. A change in SPADI score of at least 13.2–23.1/100 (or 43% of individual baseline values) indicates a minimal clinically important difference (MCID) [33, 41, 42].

Simple Shoulder Test

The Simple Shoulder Test (SST) is a (patient)self-reported questionnaire with 12 items that aims to evaluate the functional status of a patient with a shoulder problem. The SST was developed to assess the outcome of various shoulder surgeries but can also be used to evaluate shoulder function in nonoperative cases, such as the effectiveness of physical therapy. The SST is a brief and easy-to-administer questionnaire [43]. The MDC95 (0–100 range) was reported at 32.3, and the MCID ranged from 17.1 to 25 [41].

Western Ontario Rotator Cuff Index

The Western Ontario Rotator Cuff Index (WORC) can be specifically used to assess the status of the rotator cuff. This self-reported questionnaire consists of 21 items and measures the quality of life in patients with rotator cuff pathology [44]. The WORC assesses five dimensions (pain, sport/recreation, work, daily living, and emotions), with three to six questions per domain, all measured on a VAS scale. The total WORC score ranges from 0 (best) to 2100 (worst), which corresponds to 21 items × 100 mm. The MCID is estimated to be 300 [45].

Disabilities of the Arm, Shoulder, and Hand Questionnaire

The Disabilities of the Arm, Shoulder, and Hand (DASH) questionnaire is a self-reported questionnaire with 30 questions. The score ranges from 0 to 100, with 0 indicating no disability and 100 being the worst score. The MDC95 and MCID are both 10 points on average [32, 46–48].

In addition to the classic DASH questionnaire, you can also use the shortened version, the QuickDASH. It contains 11 instead of 30 questions and addresses symptoms over the past week. There are also two optional sections: sports/music and work. As with the classic DASH, a higher score indicates more symptoms and/or limitations. Both the DASH and QuickDASH are assessed using a five-point Likert scale. The MDC90 and MCID are on average 11.1 and 8 points, respectively [38].

DASH

QuickDASH

Western Ontario Shoulder Instability Index

The Western Ontario Shoulder Instability Index (WOSI) has proven to be reliable, valid, and responsive for patients with shoulder instability, covering four domains. The WOSI is a 21-item questionnaire divided into 4 domains: physical symptoms, sport/recreation/work function, lifestyle function, and emotional well-being. The scores range from no complaints (score 0) to severe complaints (score 100). The WOSI has an MDC95 of 23 points [49]. The MCID is 10% [50].

Oxford Shoulder Instability Score

The Oxford Shoulder Instability Score (OSIS) is a 12-item questionnaire with 5 response categories for each question. Answers are scored from 0 to 4, and the total score ranges from 0 (most impaired) to 48 (least impaired). The MCID (in patients undergoing arthroscopic Bankart repair for shoulder instability) is 8.6 [51].

The Western Ontario Osteoarthritis of the Shoulder Index

The Western Ontario Osteoarthritis of the Shoulder (WOOS) index measures the impact of shoulder osteoarthritis on a patient's quality of life. It consists of 19 items divided into 4 domains: physical symptoms, sport/recreation, work, and lifestyle. Each item is scored on a 100-point visual analog scale, with a total score ranging from 0 (best) to 1900 (worst), typically converted to a percentage. WOOS is recognized as a reliable and valid tool; however, we must acknowledge a large lack of orthopedic literature regarding the psychometric properties of the WOOS [52–56]. For patients with glenohumeral osteoarthritis treated with an anatomical total shoulder arthroplasty, the MCID value for the Danish version of the WOOS is 12.3 points [57].

Oxford Shoulder Score

The Oxford Shoulder Score (OSS) is a useful questionnaire originally developed for use in patients after shoulder surgery. The questionnaire consists of 12 questions that assess pain and limitations over the past 4 weeks in the patient's personal and professional life. A higher score indicates worse functioning and more pain. The OSS is scored from 12 to 60 points. Both the MCID and MDC95 are 6 points [43, 58].

The American Shoulder and Elbow Surgeons Standardized Assessment

The American Shoulder and Elbow Surgeons Standardized Assessment (ASES) evaluates shoulder pain and functional limitations [59]. The ASES consists of two subscales: one pain item scored from 0 to 10 and ten functional items using a 4-point Likert scale. Both pain and function contribute equally to the overall score, which ranges from 0 (worst) to 100 (best). While a systematic review has confirmed the ASES as a reliable and valid tool, further research is required to assess its responsiveness over time in various contexts [32]. The MDC90 is 10.5, and the MCID is 15.5 points (15% total change) [58].

Questionnaires Focusing on Psychosocial Experience

Fear-Avoidance Beliefs Questionnaire

The Fear-Avoidance Beliefs Questionnaire (FABQ) assesses pain-related fear in patients with shoulder pain [60]. The FABQ consists of 16 items, each scored from 0 to 6, where the patient indicates the degree to which they agree with the statement. Higher scores on the FABQ indicate greater pain and limitations experienced by the patient. The maximum score is 96.

Tampa Scale of Kinesiophobia

The Tampa Scale of Kinesiophobia (TSK) assesses self-reported fear of movement [61]. It consists of two subscales: avoidance of activities influenced by fear of pain or injury and beliefs about a serious cause of their condition. The TSK comprises 17 items, with a total score ranging from 17 to 68, where a higher score indicates a greater degree of fear of movement.

Pain Catastrophizing Scale

The Pain Catastrophizing Scale (PCS) assesses the extent of catastrophic thinking, primarily focusing on rumination, magnification, and feelings of helplessness [62]. Rumination refers to the tendency to dwell repeatedly on negative thoughts or past events. The PCS consists of 13 items, with a total score range of 0 to 52. Each item is scored on a five-point scale.

Questionnaire Focusing on Quality of Life

For various reasons, it is important to administer a generic health status questionnaire (generic PROMs) to a patient with shoulder pain. These questionnaires are designed to measure a wide range of health aspects, including physical, psychological, and social dimensions. This approach provides insight into overall health, well-being, and *quality of life* (QoL). The results from a generic questionnaire offer a comprehensive evaluation of the patient's health status, helping to better understand the impact of the illness or condition on different domains of life. Generally, these types of questionnaires tend to be somewhat less responsive compared to joint-specific questionnaires.

In addition to benefiting the therapist by providing a better understanding of the patient's overall health, these questionnaires also offer advantages for researchers and policymakers. By having patients complete generic questionnaires, these stakeholders can gain insights into the broader impact of health issues on society and develop interventions aimed at improving general health and quality of life.

EuroQol 5 L-5D

The EuroQol 5L-5D (EQ-5D) is a standardized questionnaire that assesses five dimensions of health: mobility, self-care, daily activities, pain and discomfort, and anxiety and depression. Each domain can be rated across five levels of severity: no problems, slight problems, moderate problems, severe problems, and extreme problems. This questionnaire can be used alongside the SF-36 to create a profile of a patient's health status. Additionally, the EQ-5D includes a VAS, where individuals can rate their current health status on a scale from 0 to 100, with 0 representing the worst imaginable health and 100 representing the best imaginable health.

The EQ-5D is easy to complete and can be used free of charge (after registration) in clinical practice. There is also a version for children (EQ-5D-Y). The EQ-5D demonstrates good reliability and validity and moderate responsiveness when used in orthopedic conditions of the upper extremity [63].

Short-Form Health Survey 36

The Short-Form Health Survey (SF-36) is a widely used questionnaire designed to measure health-related quality of life and is comparable to the RAND-36. It contains 36 questions covering eight domains of health and well-being: physical functioning, physical limitations, bodily pain, general health, vitality, social functioning, emotional limitations, and mental health. Each domain is scored on a scale from 0 to 100, with higher scores indicating better health-related quality of life.

The SF-36 can be used to assess the impact of a diseases, treatments, or interventions on both physical and mental health, as well as to compare the health status of different populations. It is intended to examine the various subdomains of the SF-36 individually rather than provide a single total score. Similar to the EQ-5D, the SF-36 is less responsive than shoulder-specific questionnaires. Further research is needed to establish the MCIDs and MDCs in shoulder populations. Additionally, it is worth noting that scoring the SF-36 is not so straightforward.

6 Screening

When a patient presents with shoulder pain, the first step is to screen the patient. This process goes beyond just considering whether the patient has direct access to physical therapy. Direct access refers to the patient's right to be examined and treated by a therapist without first consulting a physician. Even without direct access, patients may present with yellow and red flags, which could indicate the need for reassessment.

Screening should be conducted both with and without direct access. In a small portion of our patients with shoulder complaints, the symptoms may appear to have a musculoskeletal origin, but a serious underlying pathology could still be present. Rapid diagnosis is essential for the best outcome. Using these so-called red flags, the clinician can rule out these serious conditions [64].

Screening is also important due to accelerated discharge from hospitals following surgical procedures. Therefore, therapists need to be vigilant for signs of post-operative complications. This means that, based on the patient's medical history and basic physical shoulder examination, we aim to form a general impression with an eye on possible red or yellow flags.

To ensure that nothing is overlooked within the screening framework, you can have the patient fill out a questionnaire about their health history before the initial examination. As a therapist, you then review this questionnaire, paying special attention to any risk factors or red flags that could warrant further investigation during history taking. Indeed, a thorough patient history can significantly guide you toward the need for more specific screening questions or tests. Finally, the therapist gathers all the information from the patient history and physical examination to determine whether the issue that brought the patient to the clinic can be treated there.

It is important to distinguish the screening process from the diagnostic process. The screening process comes first and is separate from the diagnostic process. Diagnosis is a process in which observed data is translated into a clinical picture, identifying anatomical or functional impairments, potential activity limitations, or participation restrictions, as well as mapping out factors that promote or hinder recovery. The screening process, on the other hand, primarily involves identifying

F. Struyf, *Shoulder Pain*, https://doi.org/10.1007/978-3-031-82228-5_6

risk factors or warning signs, without linking those risk factors to a clinical condition (i.e., it is not medical diagnosis). However, being alert to risk factors is not limited to the initial screening process; it also continues during the diagnostic process and any follow-up sessions.

Yellow Flags

Yellow flags are psychosocial factors that can influence a patient's shoulder pain. Questionnaires have been developed to identify these yellow flags. Examples include a passive coping style, pain catastrophizing, fear of movement, and general psychological issues. All of these can negatively impact rehabilitation. Yellow flags do not necessarily prevent therapy, but they can affect the outcome of the treatment or the way it is administered. Elevated scores on the Tampa Scale of Kinesiophobia and the Fear-Avoidance Beliefs Questionnaire have been associated with longer recovery times, chronic symptoms, and loss of work in patients with shoulder pain. As therapists, we are well trained to treat patients with yellow flags, but it may also be appropriate to refer the patient to other healthcare providers for further treatment.

Red Flags

A red flag indicates a warning signal due to risk factors for a serious underlying pathology. A symptom with a red flag therefore requires immediate attention. This is done by asking further screening questions and/or conducting tests or by making an appropriate referral. In general, we distinguish between general and specific red flags.

Symptoms that occur bilaterally, such as pain, numbness, and tingling, or symptoms that suggest the presence of a systemic disease, are always a cause for concern and warrant further investigation. Systemic symptoms include fever, unexplained sweating, nausea, fatigue, pallor, vomiting, diarrhea, unexplained weight loss, dizziness, and fainting. These are not specific to the shoulder and are therefore described as general red flags. Such symptoms, while independent of the location of the complaints, can still warrant further medical investigation.

Specific red flags have a specific relationship with the shoulder. For example, a history of cancer is always a red flag. Breast and lung cancers are the two most common types that metastasize to the shoulder and are associated with the presence of a frozen shoulder. As you can see, specific red flags can also be non-region specific.

Heart conditions can also cause shoulder pain, particularly in patients over the age of 50 or those with a (close) family history of heart disease. Patients with a history of angina, heart attack, or cardiac surgery have an increased likelihood of heart-related shoulder pain, and these signs should be considered a warning to the therapist about the potential need for further medical evaluation. It has also been suggested that pain in the shoulder region can be caused by problems in the stomach, liver, heart, gallbladder, pancreas, lungs, spleen, and ovaries.

To identify red flags, we primarily rely on the patient's medical history and the basic physical shoulder examination. We aim to determine whether the symptoms are related to a musculoskeletal issue or a serious underlying condition that requires further investigation. Recognizing these red flags is crucial when a patient presents with shoulder pain (Table 6.1).

Table 6.1 Red flags for shoulder complaints

Possible condition	History and examination findings
Tumor [65]	History of cancer
	Cancer symptoms (unexplained weight loss, pain independent of load, and unexplained fatigue)
	Unexplained mass (whether painful or not), swelling, or deformity
	Pain is described as dull and constant, independent of movement
Inflammatory conditions (polymyalgia rheumatica, rheumatoid arthritis, (pseudo-) gout, lupus, etc.) [66, 67]	Bilateral symptoms
	Pain at rest
	(Possible) fever
	General malaise
	Weight loss
	Fatigue
	Reduced mobility
Infection [65]	Red skin
	Fever
	General malaise
Fracture or unreduced dislocation [65]	Obvious trauma
	Convulsions
	Acute limiting pain
	Acute loss of mobility
	Loss of normal shape
Neurological injury [65]	Unexplained sensory or motor deficit
Visceral condition [65]	Pain that cannot be provoked by mechanical loading of the shoulder
	Pain or symptoms due to physical exhaustion or respiratory load
	Pain associated with gastrointestinal symptoms
	Scapular pain associated with the intake of fatty foods

When Is Medical Advice Required?

Medical advice or referral is required when a clear movement disorder cannot be identified or when the findings do not correspond to a neuromuscular or musculoskeletal problem. Additionally, if the therapist observes any red flags—such as unexplained symptoms, sudden loss of function, or signs of a serious underlying condition—they should exercise caution and refer the patient for medical evaluation. It is important to note that the therapist should keep in mind that a referral from a physician may be part of the medical differential diagnosis. The physician might refer the patient to a therapist to determine whether therapy will be beneficial or not. If the therapist does not have this information, they may end up sending the patient back to the physician.

► When you, as a therapist, observe red flags, report them to the physician and ask for their opinion on how to manage the situation.

The Patient History

7

As a clinician, you strive to provide optimal care. However, that optimal care should also be evident along the journey the patient takes to get to that care. A positive first impression can build trust, create a lasting impact, and serve as the foundation for the relationship that follows.

The manner in which a patient schedules their appointment can already influence their perception of care. If they feel dismissed over the phone and sense that the receptionist is rushed or uninterested, they may already feel disappointed by the lack of personal care they have received. This may also cause the patient to worry that it reflects the care they will receive, and such expectations can have an impact on the final outcome [68]. A negative first impression could weaken the patient-provider relationship. However, when the patient is greeted professionally and the administrative staff take the time to be friendly and attentive, this caring and professional interaction leaves a positive impression, helping the patient feel confident that they made the right choice for their health.

> ► Try to ensure that making an appointment is a simple process, unhurried, patient focused, professional, and caring.

In the Waiting Room

The waiting room is a unique space that can serve many purposes beyond just waiting and watching the clock. Following the first impression, the waiting room acts as an extension of that experience. The patient still has not seen or heard you, so they continue to form their opinion based on the waiting room. Ideally, a waiting room should convey professionalism and further reassure the patient that they made the right choice. It also presents an opportunity to provide initial information and education, such as through flyers or short videos on a television screen. These videos

F. Struyf, *Shoulder Pain*, https://doi.org/10.1007/978-3-031-82228-5_7

could highlight the benefits of physical activity and exercise, the importance of sleep, stress reduction, drinking less alcohol, or quitting smoking.

Additionally, the waiting room is an ideal place to gather more information about the patient. Patients can begin filling out one or more (generic) questionnaires, unless the questionnaire requires assistance. This allows them to provide details about other conditions, medications, and their medical history, as well as answer questions related to lifestyle factors like sleep, smoking, diet, and physical activity.

The First Meeting

At the very first meeting, I introduce myself as Filip Struyf, physical therapist. I keep it informal to ensure that the patient feels comfortable enough to share their story honestly. Introducing myself as Professor Struyf would not help this process at all. You can invite the patient to call you by your first name. Then, ask the patient how they would like to be addressed, and use that form consistently. Start by asking a question that has nothing to do with their complaint, such as "Was it easy for you to get here?" or "Did you have any trouble with the rain?" This shows that you are interested in the person themselves and that you care about more than just their shoulder.

► Do you have a report to finish? Then complete it before seeing the patient. Make sure your focus is entirely on them, not on your emails, smartphone, or anything happening outside your consultation room. In short, focus on the patient.

Even before the patient enters your consultation room, they may have concerns that could limit them in telling their story. The patient might be anxious, wondering whether the physician or therapist will take them seriously. Some patients may also question whether factors such as their ethnicity, religion, skin color, body shape, lifestyle choices, or gender will affect how they are approached by the healthcare provider. These fears are real and are often heightened if they have already seen multiple providers who offered different explanations for their problem.

The patient may also be anxious about the outcomes of the consultation, such as potential injections, manipulations, or surgery, or they might fear that their pain will not go away. They might be worried about travel time and waiting periods, feeling rushed during the visit. The patient could be nervous and uncertain about what will happen during the clinical visit. The list of fears can go on. You can alleviate their concerns by explaining what will happen, from the interview to the examination and the discussion afterward.

► Be aware that your patient may have various fears and remember that the most important person in the consultation is not the healthcare provider, but the patient, who was brave enough to seek help.

The Story of the Patient

Many conditions follow a characteristic pattern that can be recognized during history taking. Based on this, you can form an initial hypothesis. The patient history is therefore an interview in which you establish the patient's medical history based on their own memories. Through this interview, the healthcare provider gains a more specific understanding of the early hypotheses. All domains of the International Classification of Functioning, Disability, and Health (ICF) are mapped out during this process. Recovery-enhancing and recovery-inhibiting factors, both personal and contextual, are also important.

A good history taking requires, on the one hand, knowledge of pathophysiology, enabling the recognition, association, and comparison of symptoms with theoretical probabilities and improbabilities. At this stage, the healthcare provider is seeking information about the patient's perceived health problem. These hypotheses will guide further examination, which is carried out in the next phase.

On the other hand, the patient's experience of the complaint and how they cope with it are also important. The interaction with personal and environmental factors plays a crucial role. It is not just about explaining the symptoms in anatomical or medical terms but also about understanding the complaint in a broader context, namely, how the patient experiences their illness and how they deal with it. This is why the patient history is sometimes referred to as the "story of the patient."

No story can ever tell everything that could be said; there are always gaps. The story the patient tells is only a part of the whole. However, if we give the patient the space to tell their story, it is likely that the patient's experience of their complaint will surface clearly. If we constantly interrupt the patient and only ask closed questions, important details may go unnoticed.

> ► It should be clear that not only what the patient says is important but also how they say it. Is their body language telling us something? So pay close attention.

How Do We Let the Patient Tell Their Story?

Living with persistent shoulder pain can be accompanied by feelings of depression, anxiety, isolation, and uncertainty [69]. This is especially true for unexplained pain. Sometimes, patients struggle to find the right words, and in such cases, the use of metaphors can help, particularly when we want to convey human experiences that are the hardest to express. Pain is one such experience. When patients try to describe their pain using a metaphor, we should allow and acknowledge this as a way to build a safe bridge to express their emotions. Patients often lack the jargon or vocabulary to explain how they feel. But if we give these patients the time and space to describe their experiences, they will often show creativity and clarify how they feel through a metaphor.

Using metaphors is not only helpful for expressing feelings in words, but it also provides a shared way of communicating that you, as a healthcare provider, can use in further questioning. Additionally, recognizing metaphors demonstrates empathy for the patient. These metaphorical expressions can help us create some structure within the chaos of an uncertain pain experience.

Let us take a closer look at what patient history has to offer. For developing an effective treatment plan, a thorough and clear history taking is absolutely essential. From a good patient history, a well-considered clinical examination can be conducted, aiming to confirm the information obtained during history taking.

What Questions Should I Ask?

Start by asking one or more questions that are not related to the shoulder. Then you explain how the consultation will proceed and ask for the reason for the visit. To avoid the patient focusing solely on their shoulder, which might cause us to miss crucial information about the context of their problem, you might want to open the conversation with a general question. Think of something like "Please tell me your story, what is the problem?" or "How can I help you?" These questions are more person centered and allow you to listen to what is most important to the individual. When the patient begins to speak, it is important not to ask for clarification and to allow them to finish their initial sentences without interruption. By not interrupting, patients feel more valued and recognize that their concerns matter to you. After they finish their initial sentences, thank the patient for sharing their concerns and proceed with other relevant questions.

The patient history usually consists of four or five parts: administrative, specific, (if pain is present: pain history), additional, and social history.

Administrative Patient History

An administrative patient history is the first part of history taking. It involves gathering the patient's administrative and demographic information. This data is important for recording and identifying the patient in the medical file, as well as assessing the pre-odds of developing shoulder problems. Demographic details such as age, gender, occupation, and sports participation can offer valuable insights into the patient's risk factors for shoulder disorders. For instance, certain age groups may be more prone to degenerative conditions like rotator cuff tears, while athletes or individuals in manual labor jobs might be at higher risk for acute injuries or overuse syndromes. Family history of joint problems may also help identify hereditary risks. Typical questions that can be asked during the administrative patient history include name, date of birth, contact details, medication use, referring physician (if any), insurance information, medical history, age, gender, sports, occupation, hobbies, previous surgeries, family history, etc. At this stage, you can also begin assessing the patient's request for help.

Specific Patient History

In the specific patient history, the patient's request for help is explored in greater depth, along with further details about functional problems and the course of the condition. Here, you gather specific information about the complaint, the symptoms, and the course of the condition. The specific patient history is crucial because it enables you, as a healthcare provider, to better understand the patient's symptoms and complaints, make a differential diagnosis, plan an appropriate treatment, and evaluate progress.

The following questions can be asked:

- What is the location of the complaint?
- When did the complaints start?
- How has the complaint evolved over time?
- Does the patient experience sensory disturbances?
- Does the patient hear any sounds when performing a movement?
- Are the complaints dependent on movement or posture?
- Let the patient describe the complaint themselves, without providing too many prompts.
- Was there an accident? If yes:
  - What type of accident was it? (a fall, throwing motion, lifting, fighting, etc.)
  - What did you feel happen during the accident? (pain, dislocation, click, crack, swelling, etc.)
  - Can you describe what the arm did during the accident (mechanism of injury)?
  - Where did the accident occur? (at home, during exercise, at work, during a certain sport, on the motorcycle, etc.)
- Have you received any treatments for your complaint? If yes:
  - Medication?
  - Physical therapy?
  - Surgery?
  - Injections?
  - Complementary medicine?
- What are any limitations in activities and participation problems?

Pain History

The pain history is, of course, only applicable when the patient is experiencing pain. Pain is one of the most common complaints for which patients seek help. Before discussing various typical shoulder conditions, it is important to consider the types of pain that the patient may report. It is evident that pain is an unpleasant sensation that usually makes the patient think of tissue damage. In a general sense, acute pain warns us of danger, while chronic pain can facilitate the healing of an injury. However, when patients think of pain, they most often think of suffering.

The intensity of pain depends on various internal and external factors. The same stimulus can be experienced in unique ways by different people and under different circumstances. Even within the same person, the same stimulus may be perceived in various ways at different times.

However, most shoulder pain will be of nociceptive origin. This means that there is a local injury (e.g., to the tendon, ligaments, or muscles) that activates the pain receptors or nociceptors through mechanical (such as pressure or stretching) or chemical means (such as inflammation). Nociceptors are free nerve endings that respond to painful stimuli. These stimuli are converted into electrical impulses that are transmitted through our peripheral nervous system to our central nervous system, where they are recognized as pain. The initial sensation of pain arises in the thalamus. They will then activate an emotional response to pain via the limbic system and proceed to the cerebral cortex, where the pain is perceived and interpreted.

There are two types of nerve fibers that conduct pain: Aδ—and C-fibers. The large Aδ-fibers produce sharp, well-localized pain. This is the type of pain you feel when a needle pierces your skin or when you grab a hot cooking pot. These fibers transmit the signal very quickly, allowing your brain to react faster than your perception of pain. For instance, you will withdraw your hand from a hot stove before you even fully feel the pain. After this initial pain signal via the Aδ-fibers, the C-fibers are also activated. However, the conduction of pain signals through C-fibers is much slower. The pain will be described by the patient as dull or burning and is less well localized. At the ends of these nerve fibers are various receptors, primarily opioid receptors. Moreover, there are inactive or "dormant" receptors that can be "awakened" by, for example, inflammation.

In summary, pain occurs in two phases: first through the fast-conducting Aδ-fibers and then through the C-fibers. Various factors can influence pain, such as endogenous opioids (e.g., endorphins) that can inhibit pain impulses by affecting chemical mediators like histamine, substance P, bradykinin, and acetylcholine. Everyone has different levels of endorphins, so pain is experienced differently by each person. Psychological factors, like the threat of pain and expectations of relief, can also affect spinal pain transmission and change how pain is perceived.

When there is an injury to the nerve tissue, there is a chance of neuropathic pain, also known as neuralgia. This can be caused by external forces such as compression, inflammation, or even by an infection. Damage can also result from chemotherapy, pressure from tumors, surgical procedures, diabetes, and so on. Damage to a part of the nerve can lead to a local inflammatory response and thus pain. The pain may also be felt further distally along the course of the affected nerve. These pain signals do not serve a specific function other than to alert the patient that something is wrong with the nerve. Much neuropathic pain is chronic in nature. The patient experiences the pain as shooting or burning. They may also feel tingling or a sensation of electric shocks.

Nociplastic pain (central sensitization) is a term used to describe a form of chronic pain that arises from changes in the nervous system. It is a type of pain where the pain experience is amplified due to alterations in our neural pathways. As a result, pressure pain thresholds are lowered, and the patient reports pain more quickly. An example of this is allodynia. This involves the nerve becoming more sensitive, causing even mild or normal stimuli are experienced as painful. This can lead to persistent pain that does not respond well to conventional painkillers or treatments. Persistent pain thus shows a plasticity that can modulate both peripheral and central pain signals. In the case of chronic pain, it either amplifies the pain signals or makes them hypersensitive.

The location is often used to identify the exact site of the complaint. This also allows you to narrow down the possible causes. This is particularly useful for finding the source of nociception. Unfortunately, the site of the pain is not always the site of the injury, so pain can be very vague. Consider rotator cuff-related complaints that cause pain in the broad region of the deltoid muscle.

Additionally, referred pain is also possible. This type of pain is felt in the shoulder but originates from a completely different region of the body. Referred pain is usually the result of a misinterpretation in our brain, and it can be felt in a specific dermatome. Local provocation tests will typically be negative. The intensity of the pain the patient feels is difficult to assess. To estimate the intensity, visual analog scales are used to compare the pain to the most severe pain the patient has ever experienced. A verbal numerical scale is also an option. We have explored this further in the chapter on questionnaires.

The duration of the complaints is somewhat easier to measure. This allows us to distinguish between acute and chronic complaints. This distinction is often based on time. In summary, pain can be acute, chronic, or intermittent. Intermittent pain occurs when the patient experiences an acute flare-up of a chronic complaint. Pain that lasts longer than 3 months is considered chronic.

Regarding the nature of pain, we refer to how the patient describes it. This allows us to distinguish between pain of neural origin (shooting, burning, tingling) and pain of vascular origin (pulsing, dull).

Social Patient History

During the social patient history, you gather information about the social and environmental factors that may influence the patient's complaint. Here, you ask questions about living and work situations, as well as lifestyle. Consider questions such as Do you have children? What social network do you have? Do you receive any help at home? Do you live alone or with a partner/children? Do you experience stress at work? Do you enjoy your work? Do you pay attention to diet and physical activity? and so on. Then, have the patient indicate any other complaints they may have. This can be an open question or, perhaps better, a checklist of various general, cardiovascular, pulmonary, metabolic, lymphatic, musculoskeletal, gastrointestinal, neurological, urological, and psychological conditions. The patient only needs to review and check off any items that apply. This approach gives you greater insight into the broader context in which the patient functions.

The last decades, it has indeed become increasingly clear that assessing lifestyle plays an important role in understanding the clinical picture of the patient. Lifestyle is a general term for the way a person lives. Some individuals have more control over their lifestyle than others. We typically refer to a lifestyle as healthy or unhealthy. Smoking, unhealthy eating (and drinking), lack of physical activity, poor sleep, obesity, and mental stress are all factors that contribute to an unhealthy lifestyle. The consequences of these factors often, but not exclusively, manifest as metabolic problems, such as hyperlipidemia, hyperglycemia, hypertension, and obesity.

Although we are increasingly seeing lifestyle factors associated with musculoskeletal complaints, including shoulder pain, it remains difficult to pinpoint a causal relationship. For example, a patient presents with shoulder pain and depression. This leads to a chicken-and-egg discussion. Nevertheless, there is growing evidence that lifestyle factors are at least associated with the complaints. Sometimes they may be the cause, sometimes the effect of the complaint, and sometimes they have an influencing force. In any case, it seems increasingly important to understand these factors so that they can potentially be linked to the clinical picture and addressed in the recovery process.

Education about lifestyle and support for behavior change are well-known strategies for patients with conditions like metabolic syndrome, but they could also be important for patients with musculoskeletal complaints. Some of these lifestyle factors may even underlie the musculoskeletal complaint and should therefore receive as much attention as a metabolic problem.

It is very possible that psychosocial factors are risk factors for the development of shoulder pain. Or do they only influence the experience of pain? Psychosocial factors can pose a barrier to recovery, potentially leading the patient into chronicity or keeping them in it. When a patient experiences improvement, it does not necessarily indicate a change in biomechanics or structure. Expectations for recovery and expectations of a particular intervention can also affect the final outcome of treatment [70–73]. Patients who expect a good outcome often achieve better results.

There is considerable evidence that the prognosis of chronic shoulder pain is influenced by psychosocial factors [70, 74, 75]. For instance, patients who tend to catastrophize often have a worse prognosis [74], and chronic or recurrent shoulder pain in some patients is associated with symptoms of depression [76]. Additionally, patients who show a high degree of self-efficacy and expect a positive treatment outcome generally recover better [70]. This may involve how patients cope with pain and their ability to control it on their own.

The relationship between psychological stress and cardiovascular diseases is well-known. However, there also appears to be a strong association between an increased risk of cardiovascular conditions and the presence of rotator cuff tendinopathy [77]. Pro-inflammatory cytokines play a role in this process. In response to psychological stress, our body produces these pro-inflammatory cytokines. During chronic low-grade inflammation, these cytokines are affected, leading to disrupted production of serotonin and dopamine, which influence our mood [78]. Both are neurotransmitters that contribute to a sense of well-being. The relationship between chronic low-grade inflammation and depression seems to go both ways: chronic inflammation appears to increase the likelihood of depression, and, conversely, stress or continuous exposure to stress tends to increase chronic inflammation [79, 80].

When we think of social factors, we often consider the support patients receive from family and friends, how well they adhere to the therapist's treatment programs, and their work situation. How family and friends perceive the patient's complaint also turns out to be important. Family and friends are very close to the patient and can strongly influence how the patient thinks about, for example, returning to work. It is not that difficult to warn a patient about all the potential harm that could occur if they return to work, thereby instilling fear and creating dependence.

► The opposite can also be present: a supportive and encouraging environment. In that sense, it can sometimes be useful to also ask the patient about what the family and friends would think of the chosen approach.

It also appears that the relationship between patient and therapist is a very important factor. The patient must be able to trust the therapist, and the therapist, in turn, must show a clear interest in the patient's needs. With this, the beliefs of the therapist are essential. The beliefs and insights of patients often mirror those of their therapists. For example, therapists who adopt a very biomedical approach appear to be more hesitant about returning to work. For therapists with a more biopsychosocial approach, the opposite is true [81, 82]. It is clear that, as clinicians, we need to be aware of any psychosocial factors that could negatively impact the shoulder complaint. Only in this way can we achieve the best outcome for the patient.

Additional Patient History

During the final part of the patient history, you gather information that has not yet been addressed or where additional details are needed based on previous answers. Think of unaddressed comorbidities such as diabetes or obesity or habits related to sleep, smoking, or alcohol use.

Type 2 diabetes mellitus (DM) is a chronic disease characterized by elevated blood glucose levels over an extended period. When DM remains untreated, it can cause severe long-term complications to the vascular and nervous systems. Patients with DM report twice as many musculoskeletal complaints compared to healthy controls [83], including shoulder complaints. The most frequently reported shoulder problem in DM is a frozen shoulder [84, 85]. However, DM is also associated with an increased risk of persistent rotator cuff tendinopathy [86]. Chronically elevated blood glucose levels, as measured by an increase in hemoglobin-bound glucose (HbA1c), may play a significant role in the high prevalence of shoulder and other musculoskeletal disorders in DM. Notably, there are differences in musculoskeletal abnormalities between type 1 and type 2 diabetics. Although HbA1c levels appear to be similar between type 1 and type 2 diabetes, frozen shoulder occurs significantly more often in type 2 diabetes. Thus, an increase in HbA1c levels probably cannot be used as the sole reason for the development of a frozen shoulder. Other factors, such as *advanced glycation end products* (AGEs), play a role. These AGEs are significantly more prevalent in patients with DM. It is believed that these substances affect the quality of tendon tissue through collagen *cross-linking* [87]. With a recent systematic review, we were able to demonstrate that the effects of DM are not only related to the pathogenesis of frozen shoulder [88]. Indeed, DM appears to result in reduced mobility around the shoulder and not only in patients with frozen shoulder. There is also evidence of degenerative changes in the rotator cuff in patients with DM compared to healthy individuals.

Obesity is a condition characterized by an excess of body fat. "Excess" means that there is an increased risk of health problems. You might think that excess fat, aside from putting extra stress on the joints, has little effect on our health, but nothing could be further from the truth. An excess of fat mass, or adiposity, should be considered as a functioning, dynamic organism, an organism that releases various active molecules, each with its influence on inflammation. Pro-inflammatory adipokines have already been found in subacromial bursae [89]. If the patient presents with type 2 diabetes and/or obesity, it may be important to also discuss the patient's physical activity and dietary habits. There are strong correlations between a poor diet and health problems such as obesity and type 2 diabetes. There also appears to be a clear link between chronic low-grade inflammation and the level of physical activity [90]. Physical inactivity could indeed lead to the accumulation of visceral fat mass and increased chronic low-grade inflammation [91].

We know that smoking is unhealthy and affects our lungs. But there are also important reasons to quit smoking in relation to shoulder pain. The various chemical substances inhaled through smoking cause an inflammatory response [92]. This not only leads to the development of respiratory diseases but also appears to be a risk factor for other lifestyle-related metabolic disorders, such as type 2 diabetes [92]. Smoking, and specifically nicotine, indeed increases our chronic low-grade inflammation, thereby stimulating the production of pro-inflammatory cytokines [93], and this happens to be one of the typical characteristics of the pathogenesis of frozen shoulder. And not only the glenohumeral capsule but also tendons, such as the rotator cuff, are negatively affected by this. Nicotine could lead to delayed regeneration and therefore increased degeneration of our tendon tissue, partly through tissue hypoxia [94, 95]. Hypoxia promotes the expression of pro-inflammatory cytokines and also stimulates apoptotic mediators [95]. This is why hypoxic cell damage is considered a possible cause of early tendinopathy. The natural balance between degeneration and regeneration of our rotator cuff tendons under stress is thus compromised [96].

Finally, an assessment of the patients' sleep behavior can also be important for patients with shoulder pain. It has been frequently shown that patients with rotator cuff-related conditions also experience sleep problems [97]. Our sleep provides a crucial period for recovery—psychologically, immunologically, as well as cardiovascular and neuromuscular. Therefore, a lack of sleep leads to a lack of recovery opportunity. Not coincidentally, more pain and increased chronic low-grade inflammation are observed in people with reduced sleep [98, 99]. It is clear that sleep problems are often considered a consequence of musculoskeletal complaints. For example, sleep has been found to significantly improve after rotator cuff repair surgery [100]. However, there is also evidence that poor sleep patterns can be a risk factor for the development of musculoskeletal complaints [101]. Both likely go hand in hand. If you have persistent shoulder pain, you will sleep poorly. If you sleep poorly, you will experience more shoulder pain.

► Based on this additional information, the healthcare provider can gain a better understanding of the patient, their needs, and expectations, and the request for help can be adjusted or clarified if necessary. This contributes to a personalized treatment plan and the selection of appropriate interventions.

8 Clinical Examination

The definition of clinical reasoning is a reflective process of investigation and analysis, carried out by a healthcare professional in collaboration with the patient, with the aim of understanding the patient, their context, and their clinical problem(s). This understanding is then used to shape the treatment plan of the healthcare provider.

Clinical reasoning involves the combined use of medical history, the patient's story, clinical examination, and potentially supplementary imaging or blood tests. It entails gathering and analyzing information about the patient. It is a cyclical process because the information obtained through patient history, physical examination, and follow-up consultations is continuously reassessed, and hypotheses are revised if necessary. The gathered information leads to hypotheses about the patient's problem (or multiple problems) and informs the treatment strategy.

Assessing tissue irritability is also part of the patient's clinical examination, as this data is needed to gauge the intensity and focus of the intervention. From the information collected during the examination, you should be able to gradually form an image of the possible pathology of the patient through logical and analytical reasoning. Medical imaging can provide additional information. Based on the analysis of data from the clinical examination, the clinician formulates a hypothesis. Even during treatment, it is important to continuously conduct limited assessments to evaluate the treatment's outcomes with the patient. Based on these interim evaluations, adjustments may be made to the goals to be achieved, the dosage, or the chosen interventions if necessary.

But why is clinical reasoning so important? Firstly, there is the vast variety of manifestations of a similar pathological situation, ranging from a minor injury to a multifactorial biopsychosocial tangle. As a clinician, you must be capable of conducting an extensive assessment and analysis of all biopsychosocial factors known to influence health problems.

Clinical reasoning, and thus analytical thinking, inevitably leads to cognitive errors. By practicing clinical reasoning, you can further develop it and arrive at the most probable assessment and analysis. Good clinical reasoning is not easy.

F. Struyf, *Shoulder Pain*, https://doi.org/10.1007/978-3-031-82228-5_8

You need to take a step back, think about questions you want answered, the information you find important, and the conclusions you draw while remaining critical of your own findings and analyses. Clinical reasoning is therefore more than just performing a physical examination as taught or asking questions from a checklist. Throughout this process of thinking about the patient's problems, you must also continually reflect on whether your reasoning is truly hypothesis driven. Be careful of "wishful thinking" just because you think you have recognized the pattern. Stay critical.

Clinical reasoning is thus an exciting process that will need to grow through trial and error. Know that even the greatest experts still make mistakes. These mistakes should not deter you from continuing the search with the next patient. After all, you have learned from previous situations and have taken another step closer to the ideal scenario, if such a thing as an ideal situation even exists.

Based on the data collected during the patient history, research goals are formulated before the actual examination begins. These research goals are established through visual assessment, palpation, and a basic physical examination. In this chapter, we focus on the evaluation of the shoulder girdle. However, it is crucial to recognize that the functions of the neck, torso, and even the elbow should also be evaluated, as they can significantly impact shoulder function. Musculoskeletal issues often do not exist in isolation; rather, they can be interconnected. Evaluating adjacent regions allows for a more comprehensive understanding of the patient's condition, revealing underlying factors that may contribute to shoulder pain or dysfunction. By considering the entire kinetic chain, we can develop more effective treatment plans and improve overall outcomes.

Visual Assessment

The purpose of the visual assessment is to observe and document visible changes in the patient. During the subsequent examination, you, as the practitioner, further analyze these changes and investigate their possible relationship to the patient's complaints. The assessment begins as soon as the patient enters the treatment room and continues during the basic physical shoulder examination.

► As a clinician, you always conduct a general assessment from the ventral, dorsal, and lateral views, as well as a local assessment of the affected area.

The general assessment includes several aspects. First, activities of daily living are observed, with special attention to the affected body part. Next, posture, body composition, the use of assistive devices, and overall presentation, including the patient's psychological state, are assessed. This is followed by an evaluation of the static posture, where the relationships between the spine, pelvis, and lower limbs are assessed. Finally, the shape of the skeleton and muscles is evaluated, along with the condition of the skin, nails, and (body) hair.

During the local assessment, you focus on the affected region. You carefully examine the contours of the shoulder girdle: is there any visible atrophy, discoloration, or scarring? You also pay close attention to any antalgic postures, such as an exaggerated elevation of the affected side. Furthermore, you assess any potential (sub)luxation of the acromioclavicular joint and evaluate the scapular position at rest and later during active movements. Compensatory movements of the scapula are frequently observed in combination with shoulder complaints, often defined as scapular dyskinesis.

Scapular dyskinesis refers to an alteration in the normal movement pattern of the scapula and is often observed in patients with rotator cuff-related shoulder pain. Although scapular dyskinesis can theoretically lead to a reduction of the subacromial space and result in shoulder pain, there is no conclusive evidence that this movement disorder is the cause of the pain. Various studies have shown that changes in muscle activity due to pain can also lead to scapular dyskinesis, suggesting that it is more likely an effect than a cause of possible shoulder pain.

Brief Palpation

Before and after the basic physical shoulder examination, perform a palpation, initially to assess warmth and swelling in the affected area. You can evaluate the temperature by placing the back of your hand against the patient's skin and comparing left and right. You can also locate any swelling and try to determine whether it is more likely intra-articular or extra-articular. After the basic physical shoulder examination, you can perform targeted palpation to identify sensitive areas. All of this provides insight into the current state of the complaints and the impact of movement on the condition.

Active and Passive Movement Assessment

The evaluation of mobility is an integral part of a physical examination. Mobility refers to the freedom of movement in various directions. Normal mobility is achieved when the full (pain-free) *range of motion* (ROM) is attainable in all directions, there is a normal end feel, and no abnormal resistance is experienced during passive movements. The term "end feel" refers to the sensation of resistance encountered at the end of a joint's range of motion during passive movement. A "normal end feel" indicates that the shoulder joint is functioning as expected, typically characterized by either a soft or firm end feel. When examining the shoulder, a soft end feel is common, resulting from the approximation of soft tissues—specifically, the compression of muscles that limits further movement. In some cases, you may also encounter a firm, elastic end feel due to the stretching of ligaments. A hard end feel is generally atypical for the shoulder, as it usually indicates bone-to-bone contact. An end feel described as empty (often associated with pain) or hard (which may suggest bony obstruction) can indicate potential joint issues that require further investigation.

The shoulder's joint mobility is structurally limited by intra- and extra-articular factors. Intra-articular factors include the shape of the glenohumeral joint and the joint capsule (and possibly a part of the long head of the musculus biceps brachii). Extra-articular factors include muscles, tendons, ligaments, nerves, bursae, skin, blood vessels, and so on. Active range of motion (aROM) refers to the amount of movement possible during voluntary joint movements without external assistance. Active-assisted ROM is a form of aROM where an external force (e.g., manual) is used to further complete the movement. Passive ROM (pROM) is the range of motion achieved entirely with the help of an external force, such as the therapist.

Recognizing limitations in joint mobility can assist clinicians in making working diagnoses, measuring changes in mobility, and identifying functional impairments. You assess how this load affects the symptoms. Components of this functional assessment include, for example, an active and passive functional assessment and a resistance test. All structures involved in the relevant segment are included in the functional assessment. For instance, in the case of brachialgia, you examine from the cervical and thoracic region down to the fingers.

Shoulder mobility can be assessed in various ways. In addition to visual assessment, a goniometer or inclinometer is a standard tool. A goniometer consists of a protractor-like device that can measure angles. A goniometer requires the recognition of anatomical landmarks, whereas an inclinometer uses gravity as a reference. Besides a goniometer or inclinometer, mobility can also be assessed using various questionnaires that map the patient's problems. Think of the Disabilities of the Arm, Shoulder, and Hand (DASH) questionnaire or the Shoulder Pain and Disability Index. Although these are not direct measurement tools for shoulder mobility, they are widely used patient-reported outcome measures that assess the impact of upper extremity disability, including shoulder mobility.

In combination with the standardized local anatomical examination of the shoulder joint, it is also advisable to perform a functional assessment to determine which functions are impaired and which activities are limited, in the context of the ICF. When you want to document activity limitations, have the patient perform several activities, preferably linked to the patient's story. Think of simple activities such as weight-bearing or movements related to the patient's work, hobbies, or sports. You again assess for any limitations and evaluate the presence of pain.

It is generally recommended to test anteflexion, retroflexion, abduction, external rotation (in 0 and 90 degrees of abduction), internal rotation (in 0 and 90 degrees of abduction), horizontal abduction, and horizontal adduction. Here, we will focus on some measurements of active ROM that have proven to be reliable. Both the inclinometer and the goniometer measurements have good reliability [102].

Anteflexion ROM

You can assess the active anteflexion ROM (Fig. 8.1a) with the patient either standing or sitting, which helps prevent compensatory extension of the spine. You can control this extension by providing instructions and using a wall or chair back for the patient to lean against. Then you ask the patient to actively lift the arm in the sagittal plane with the palm facing downward until the movement comes to an end. Next, you perform the measurement, for example, using an inclinometer (placed distally on the humerus, proximal to the elbow, just after the deltoid muscle insertion) or a goniometer (one arm parallel to the humerus, one arm parallel to the trunk, with the hinge at the inferior and lateral corner of the acromion) (Fig. 8.1b).

Abduction ROM

You can also assess the active abduction ROM (Fig. 8.2a) with the patient either sitting or standing. Again, you need to ensure that no lateral flexion of the spine occurs. Then you ask the patient to actively lift the arm in a frontal plane, with the thumb pointing upward toward the ceiling. Next, you perform the measurement again using an inclinometer (placed distally on the humerus, proximal to the elbow,

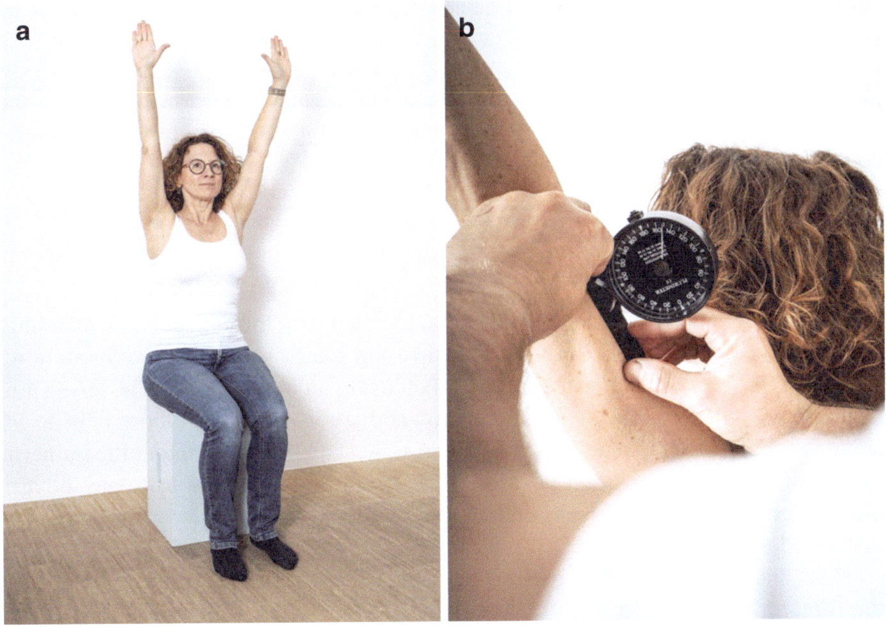

Fig. 8.1 (**a**) Active anteflexion ROM, (**b**) measurement of active anteflexion ROM with an inclinometer

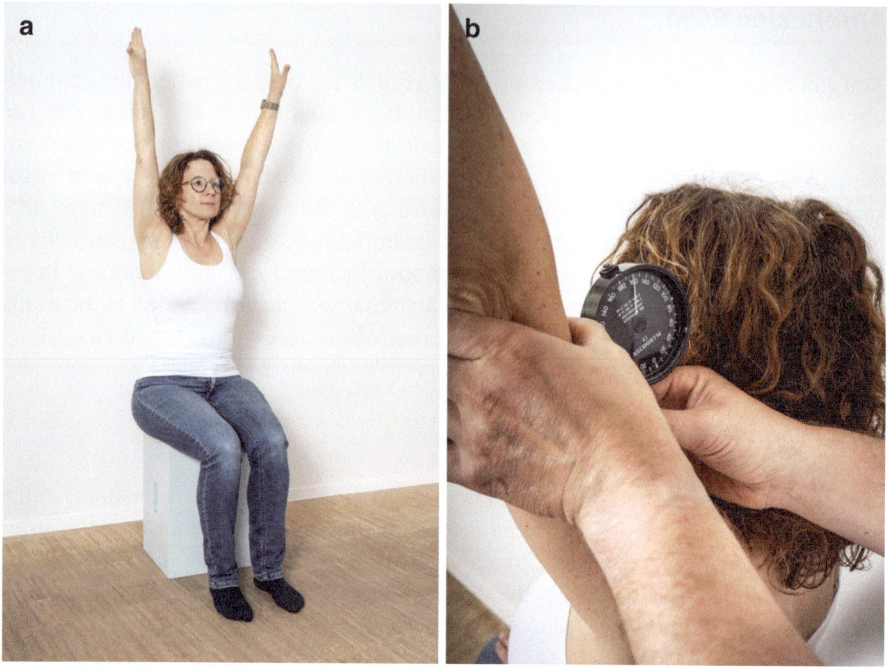

Fig. 8.2 (**a**) Active abduction ROM, (**b**) measurement of active abduction ROM with inclinometer

just after the deltoid muscle insertion) or a goniometer (one arm parallel to the humerus, one arm parallel to the trunk, with the hinge at the inferior and lateral corner of the acromion) (Fig. 8.2b).

External Rotation ROM

The active external rotation ROM (Fig. 8.3a) is tested with the patient either standing/sitting or in a supine position with the hips and knees bent to approximately 45 degrees. The latter position is necessary when using an inclinometer. The tested arm is supported on the table in 90 degrees of abduction, with the elbow bent to 90 degrees and the wrist in a neutral position. A towel can be placed under the humerus to ensure a neutral horizontal position. The patient is then asked to rotate the arm into external rotation until the end of the available mobility. The participant is instructed not to lift the lower back during this measurement.

Next, the measurement is performed using an inclinometer (placed distally on the forearm, proximal to the wrist) or a goniometer (one arm parallel to the treatment table, one arm parallel to the forearm). The measurement can be conducted with the arm in 0 degrees and in 90 degrees of abduction (Fig. 8.3b).

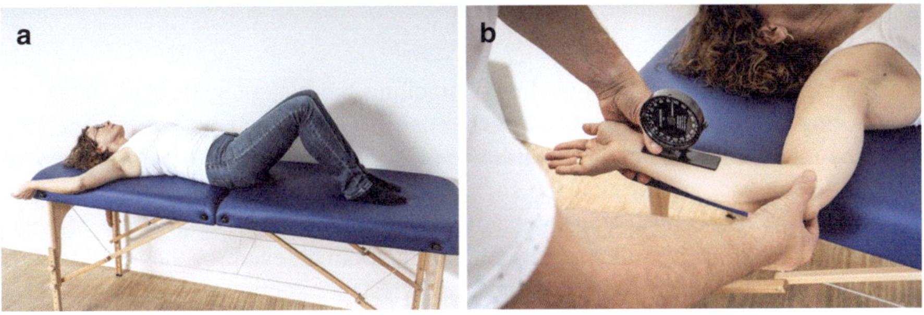

Fig. 8.3 (**a**) Active external rotation ROM, (**b**) measurement of active external rotation ROM with inclinometer

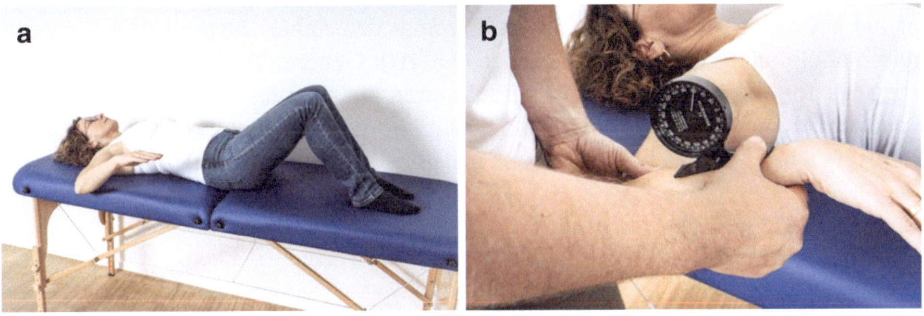

Fig. 8.4 (**a**) Active internal rotation ROM, (**b**) measurement of active internal rotation ROM with inclinometer

Internal Rotation ROM

The active internal rotation ROM (Fig. 8.4a) is tested with the patient either standing/sitting or in a supine position with the hips and knees bent to approximately 45 degrees. The latter position is necessary when using an inclinometer. The tested arm is supported on the table in 90 degrees of abduction, with the elbow bent to 90 degrees and the wrist in a neutral position. A towel can be placed under the humerus to ensure a neutral horizontal position. You then ask the patient to rotate the arm into internal rotation until the end of the available mobility, making sure that the 90-degree abduction position is maintained.

Through verbal correction, you also ensure that the scapula does not perform a protraction movement. The participant is instructed not to lift the lower back during this measurement. Next, the measurement is performed again using an inclinometer (placed distally on the forearm, proximal to the wrist) or a goniometer (one arm parallel to the treatment table, one arm parallel to the forearm). The measurement can be conducted with the arm in 0 degrees and in 90 degrees of abduction (Fig. 8.4b).

Resistance Testing

Evaluating muscle strength is useful for tracking the patient's strength status and monitoring their progress. Measurements can be performed before, during, and after the intervention. They help guide the prescribed exercise protocol. Moreover, testing muscle strength around the shoulder allows you to quantify the isometric, eccentric, and concentric capacities of the shoulder muscles. Muscle strength assessment using valid, reliable, and clinically applicable approaches could therefore be a valuable part of a comprehensive physical examination of the shoulder. In addition to strength, resistance testing can also provide insight into potential pain provocation, willingness to move, and coordination.

The methods for quantifying shoulder strength are numerous. However, to be meaningful, clinical assessment methods must be valid and reliable. Moreover, these methods provide clinicians with data to assess clinically relevant changes, one of the key values for establishing the minimal detectable change (MDC) and the minimal clinically important difference (MCID). Generally, there are three typical methods for measuring shoulder muscle strength: manual muscle tests (MMT), handheld dynamometry (HHD), and isokinetic muscle strength testing (IMST). Below is a brief overview of their pros and cons.

Manual Muscle Testing

Manual muscle tests (MMT) are widely used to clinically evaluate shoulder muscle strength. The frequent use is likely due to the ease with which the technique can be performed quickly and without cost. With MMT, the strength of the shoulder muscles can be graded as described by Hayes [103]: grade 1 indicates the absence of muscle contraction as determined by observation and palpation; grade 2 is scored when the subject is able to move the arm without gravity load; grade 3 is reported when the subject can move the arm against gravity; finally, grades 4, 4.5, and 5 are scored when the subjects can resist a load in a mid-position, defined as low, moderate, and high resistance, respectively.

However, MMT has been criticized for testing shoulder muscles due to its subjectivity and lack of reliability, as the execution of the test depends on the experience, strength, and judgment of the examiner [103–105]. The inter-rater reliability of manual muscle tests resulted in intraclass correlation coefficients (ICCs) ranging from 0.38 to 0.72 [103]. Such low levels of reliability or reproducibility are generally considered insufficient for clinical use. Additionally, low correlations have been reported between MMT and isokinetic muscle strength tests, further questioning its validity [106]. Therefore, handheld dynamometry may be a better alternative.

Handheld Dynamometry

Clinicians often use handheld dynamometry (HHD), which is easy to handle and portable, for assessing muscle strength. Hayes et al. [106] demonstrated that HHD could be performed during elevation, external rotation, internal rotation, and during the hand-behind-the-back lift-off maneuver, all in a seated position.

During elevation, the tester places the affected arm of a seated patient in 90 degrees and 30 degrees of elevation in the frontal plane with the thumb pointing medially (Fig. 8.5). The patient is asked to hold this position while the tester applies a downward force on the distal end of the forearm.

During internal or external rotation, the tester positions the affected arm in 90 degrees of elbow flexion with the thumb pointing upward and the humerus alongside the torso (Fig. 8.6a, b). The tester then applies force to the dorsal/volar side of the distal end of the forearm in the direction of external/internal rotation, while the

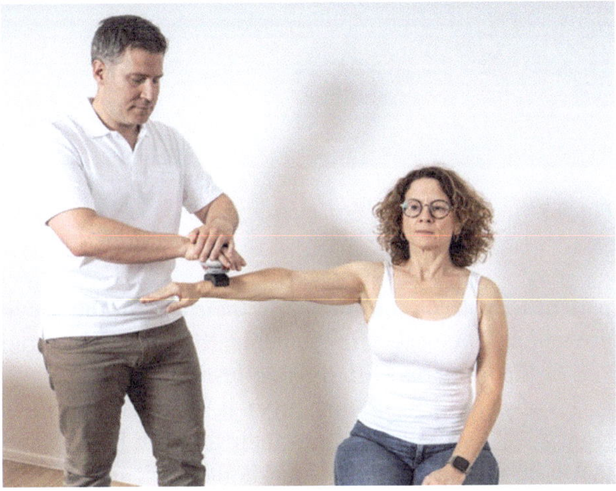

Fig. 8.5 Handheld dynamometry during elevation

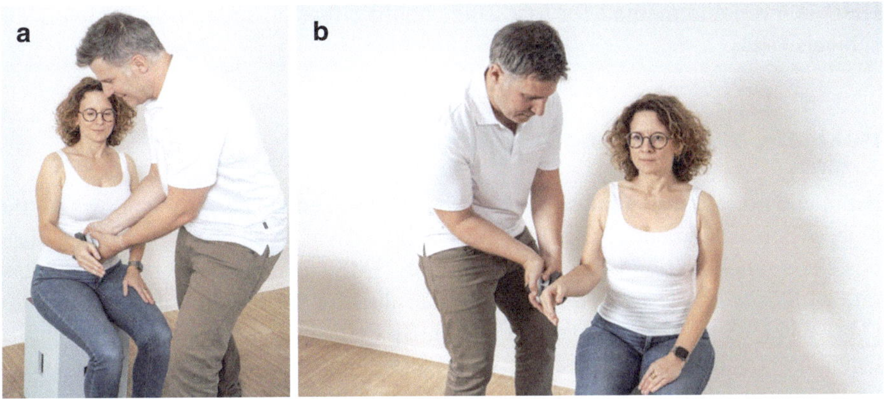

Fig. 8.6 Handheld dynamometry during internal rotation (**a**) and external rotation (**b**)

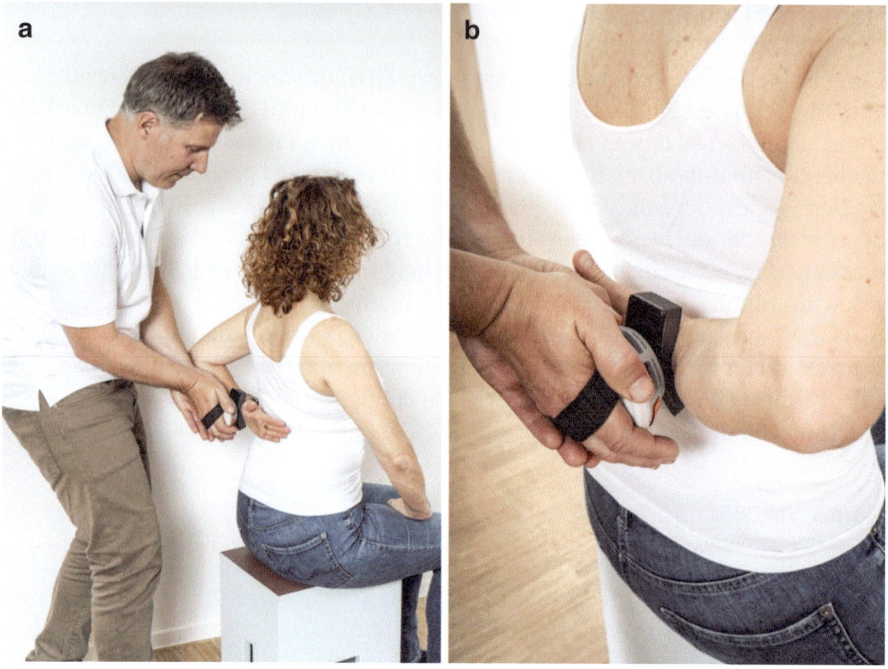

Fig. 8.7 (**a, b**) Handheld dynamometry during the lift-off maneuver

patient is instructed to maintain their arm in the previously described position. To prevent compensatory movements, the tester can provide stabilization to the distal end of the humerus with the non-testing hand.

Finally, the lift-off maneuver is used to test internal rotation muscle strength (Fig. 8.7). The patient places their forearm behind their back without making contact with the back. The patient is then asked to hold that position while the tester applies anteriorly directed resistance on the volar side of the distal forearm. The HHD is a reliable method for assessing shoulder muscle strength in symptomatic subjects [103].

Isokinetic Muscle Strength Testing

Isokinetic muscle strength testing (IMST) is recommended because it allows for the objective measurement of shoulder muscle strength and can be used to guide diagnosis and rehabilitation [107–110]. Generally, IMST is reported to be highly accurate with excellent test-retest reliability in evaluating the shoulder muscle complex [111, 112]. However, Edouard et al. [113] described differences in reliability depending on the patient's position (sitting, standing, or lying), the mode of contraction (concentric or eccentric), and the position of the shoulder. They concluded that the sitting position with 45 degrees of shoulder abduction in the scapular plane resulted in the highest reliability scores. This corresponds with the position in the scapular plane, which offers biomechanical advantages and provides the patient with maximum safety and comfort during the test. Every advantage has its disadvantage, and that applies here as well. Despite its high accuracy, IMST requires expensive equipment that takes up a lot of space, which may not be feasible for many clinicians.

The Role of Special Tests

After the basic physical shoulder examination, the most important part of the clinical assessment has already been completed. Based on these findings and assuming there are no red flags, you, as a healthcare provider, may choose to perform further clinical tests and possibly supplement them with imaging. After the screening, you also make a judgment about the involvement of the shoulder joint in the complaint. Are the symptoms attributable to a shoulder pathology or to the cervical spine? Typically, having the patient move their neck in different directions, possibly supplemented with neural tension tests, is sufficient to distinguish the origin of the complaints.

Remember that a patient may also have neck pain because of a shoulder problem. This is especially true for patients who elevate the shoulder (particularly scapular) to gain more range of motion. As a result, the upper part of the trapezius muscle can become painful and cause discomfort. However, in this case, it is not the neck causing the shoulder pain but the other way round.

Traditionally, we have tried to identify the anatomical structure responsible for the complaint. However, it is crucial to recognize that, for various reasons, this is not always possible—and, fortunately, it is not always necessary to map out an effective treatment plan. First, the shoulder is a very complex collection of structures that are not always easily distinguishable from one another. This complexity is particularly important when it comes to traumatic tears, as differentiating between the supraspinatus and infraspinatus muscles is vital; the surgical approach will vary significantly depending on which muscle is affected. However, in the case of tendinopathies or smaller tears, even if imaging reveals damage, such as hypoechoic areas on an ultrasound imaging device, the source of the complaint might still stem from another structure. Fortunately, this ambiguity does not need to cause frustration; we can often develop a conservative treatment plan even without knowing the exact origin of the complaint.

Several additional tests have been developed to identify specific shoulder conditions. These additional tests have a sensitivity, a specificity, a positive and negative predictive value, a positive and negative *likelihood* ratio, and a reliability. Moreover, there is considerable variation in the findings of these values between studies. Additionally, the gold standard against which these tests were compared often relied on imaging or direct visualization during surgery. The gold standard is therefore based on identified tissue pathology without knowing whether the pathological tissue actually caused the symptoms. In this book, we have selected tests with the highest evidence for practical usefulness.

Imaging procedures such as X-ray/CT, ultrasound, and MRI are also useful for diagnosis, as they help directly identify tissue pathology. We will discuss their value in a separate chapter on the role of imaging.

Properties of a Clinical Test

When we want to make a judgment about a patient's health condition and use tests for this purpose, we must recognize that these tests are sometimes imperfect or ambiguous. Therefore, it is important to determine the extent to which these tests can establish the likely presence or absence of a condition. Only then can we improve our decision-making using their findings.

When testing the clinimetric properties of a test, it is often compared to the gold standard for the same target condition. The term "gold standard" suggests that this initial classification is made based on a test that provides authoritative and presumably indisputable evidence of whether a condition is present or not [114]. Due to concerns about the value of these so-called gold standards, they are increasingly referred to as 'reference standards'. Based on the results of the reference standard (e.g., the MRI result of a rotator cuff tear) and the results of the clinical test, individuals are classified into one of the four cells A through D in Table 8.1.

The sensitivity, specificity, and positive and negative predictive values can be calculated from the number of individuals in each of the four cells. These properties are then expressed as percentages. It is important not to confuse the concepts of sensitivity/specificity with positive/negative predictive value. On the one hand, it is crucial for a test to have high sensitivity and high specificity. On the other hand, these values should not be used when making decisions about individual persons in screening situations. In that second situation, the use of predictive values is much more appropriate. This is explained further below.

Only when both sensitivity and specificity are very high can these concepts be useful. Here, the mnemonic SPIN and SNOUT can be helpful. SNOUT stands for Sensitive, Negative, and OUT. This means that you can very likely exclude the condition when the clinical test is negative in the case of a highly sensitive test. In the

Table 8.1 Schematic overview of the concepts of sensitivity, specificity, positive predictive value, and negative predictive value

	Positive according to reference standard	Negative according to reference standard	
Clinical test is positive	True positive A	False positive B	Positive predictive value (%) = (A/(A + B)) × 100
Clinical test is negative	False negative C	True negative D	Negative predictive value (%) = (D/(C + D)) × 100
	Sensitivity (%) = (A/(A + C)) × 100	Specificity (%) = (D/(B + D)) × 100	

case of a very sensitive test, there are likely to be almost no false negatives (cell A is high, cell C is low). High sensitivity allows you to confidently assume that people do not have the condition if their test yields a negative result. They can, therefore, be "ruled out."

SPIN stands for Specificity, Positive, and INclude. This means that you can very likely include the condition when the clinical test is positive in the case of a highly specific test. In the case of a very specific test, there are likely to be almost no false positives (cell D is high, cell B is low). High specificity allows you to confidently assume that people have the condition if their test yields a positive result. They can, therefore, be "ruled in."

But again, the mnemonic SPIN and SNOUT can only be useful when both sensitivity and specificity are very high. Moreover, this concept of SPIN and SNOUT is somewhat counterintuitive.

Sensitivity and Positive Predictive Value

The sensitivity is the fraction of true positives among those who are injured or the fraction of a group of individuals with the condition being tested that are correctly classified as injured. If all injured individuals are labeled as "injured" (meaning they receive a positive test result), the sensitivity is at its maximum: 1 (or 100%).

> Sensitivity = number of true positives/(number of true positives + number of false negatives)

A test with 100% sensitivity correctly identifies all patients with the disease. A test with 80% sensitivity detects 80% of the patients with the disease (true positives), but 20% of those with the disease remain undetected (false negatives). A high sensitivity is particularly important when the test is used to detect a serious disease (such as cancer). Tests for such conditions should be as sensitive as possible because we want to minimize the number of false negatives. Sensitivity is therefore typically described as the ability of a test to detect a truly positive result. The positive predictive value is the fraction of individuals with a positive result who indeed have the pathology (the probability of having the condition with a positive result).

The sensitivity is a useful tool, but it primarily tells us whether someone who tests positive on the reference standard also has a positive or negative clinical test. Patients typically do not walk into a doctor's office and say, "I've been diagnosed with this disease and want to know the likelihood that the tests will be positive." However, what we are practically more interested in is the question, "What if a person tests positive on the clinical test?" This is the practical translation. While sensitivity focuses on the performance of the clinical test relative to the reference standard, the positive predictive value concerns the test's usefulness in clinical practice.

This distinction is already evident when you look at Table 8.1. The sensitivity is only based on cells A and C, meaning that all individuals in the analysis must be diagnosed according to the reference standard as definitely having the condition. In determining sensitivity, no account is taken of individuals who, according to the reference standard, do not have the condition in question (cells B and D). Therefore, if we want to make a judgment based on a positive test result about who has the condition and who does not, we also need information about the data in cell B and thus calculate the positive predictive value. Simply put, the positive predictive value is the probability that people with a positive clinical test result indeed have the condition.

Specificity and Negative Predictive Value

The specificity is the fraction of true negatives among those who are not injured or the fraction of a group of individuals without the condition being tested that are correctly classified as not injured.

> Specificity = number of true negatives/(number of true negatives + number of false positives)

A test with 100% specificity will correctly identify all individuals without the disease. A test with 80% specificity correctly identifies 80% of true negatives, but 20% of individuals without the disease are incorrectly identified as positive (false positives).

The negative predictive value is the fraction of individuals with a negative result who indeed do not have the pathology (the probability of not having the condition with a negative result).

The reasoning we applied to sensitivity can now be extended to specificity and negative predictive value. Specificity is based on cells B and D. In determining specificity, no account is taken of individuals who, according to the reference standard, do have the condition. However, from a practical standpoint, we are more interested in the question, "What does it mean if a person tests negative on the clinical test?" This is where the negative predictive value becomes relevant.

Likelihood Ratios

Clinicians are quite familiar with the concepts of sensitivity, specificity, and predictive values. A less well-known but equally interesting characteristic of clinical tests is the likelihood ratios (LR). These ratios use the concepts of specificity and sensitivity to calculate the probability of a condition.

The LR indicates how much more likely a person with the condition is to have a positive test result compared to a person without the condition. The positive LR (LR+) is typically a number greater than 1, while the negative LR (LR-) is typically less than 1.

LR+ is the ratio of the probability of a positive test result in individuals with the pathology to the probability of a positive test result in individuals without the pathology. A diagnostic test becomes more informative as the LR+ increases. When a positive result is obtained with a high LR+, it is more likely that the pathology is present.

Likelihood ratio positive (LR+) = sensitivity/(1 – specificity)

LR- is the ratio of the probability of a negative test result in individuals with the pathology to the probability of a negative test result in individuals without the pathology. A diagnostic test becomes more informative as the LR- decreases (approaches zero). With a negative result and a low LR-, it is much less likely that the pathology is present.

Likelihood ratio negative (LR−) = (1 – sensitivity)/specificity

The following values are typically used for interpreting the likelihood ratio:

>10: Strong increase in the likelihood of a condition
5–10: Moderate increase in the likelihood of a condition
2–5: Small increase in the likelihood of a condition
1–2: Minimal increase in the likelihood of a condition
1: No change in the likelihood of a condition
0.5–1.0: Minimal decrease in the likelihood of a condition
0.2–0.5: Small decrease in the likelihood of a condition
0.1–0.2: Moderate decrease in the likelihood of a condition
<0.1: Large and often decisive decrease in the likelihood of a condition

How do you use these ratios in practice? Based on the medical history, and prevalence of a condition, an estimate is made of the probability of a specific shoulder condition. Let us take the example of glenohumeral instability, using the *apprehension test.* According to a study by Noorani et al. [115], the prevalence of atraumatic instability is estimated between 2% and 30% (with an average of 16%). The *apprehension test* has a sensitivity of 70% and a specificity of 96% for apprehension as the main symptom [116]. This results in an LR+ of 17.5 and an LR- of 0.31. Next, we plot the pretest probability on the *likelihood* ratios in a nomogram. As you can see, the pretest probability of 16% increases to about 76% posttest if the test is positive. If the test is negative, the estimated probability of glenohumeral instability decreases from 16% to about 6%.

As you can see, much depends on the pretest probability. We have now chosen a general prevalence. If we also consider a patient history of clicking and fear, along with a history of subluxation, our pretest probability would be closer to 30%. This would increase the posttest probability to 90%.

The nomogram (Fig. 8.8) provides a good estimate of the posttest probability of a condition. If the test is positive, we estimate this at around 76%. However, if you want more precise figures, you can also use the pretest odds. First, you convert the pretest probability into pretest odds:

Pretest probability/(1 – pretest probability) = 0.16/(1–0.16) = 0.19

Next, you calculate the posttest odds:

Pretest odds × LR+ = 0.19 × 17.5 = 3.33

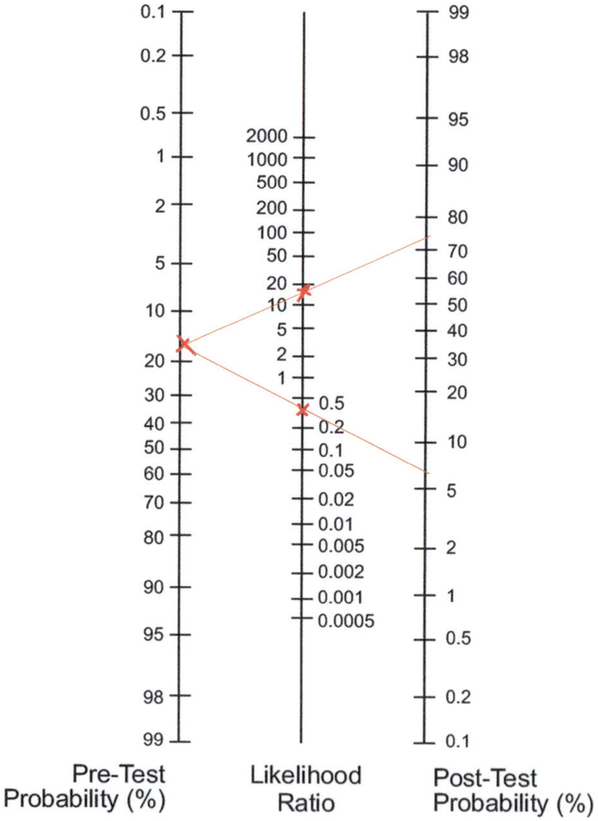

Fig. 8.8 Nomogram of Salkic 2009

Finally, we convert the posttest odds back into a posttest probability:

(Posttest odds)/(posttest odds) + 1 = 3.33/4.33 = 0.77 or 77%

In the case of a negative test, this becomes:

Pretest probability/(1 − pretest probability) = 0.16/(1 − 0.16) = 0.19
Pretest odds × LR− = 0.19 × 0.31 = 0.059
Posttest odds/(posttest odds + 1) = 0.059/1.059 = 0.056 or 5.6%

So with our 6% estimate, we were not too far off. In summary, we want to use a test with the highest possible positive *likelihood* ratio to confirm the condition and a test with the lowest possible negative *likelihood* ratio to rule out the condition. Although these concepts like sensitivity, specificity and likelihood ratios are crucial in understanding the probabilistic and stepwise nature of diagnostic reasoning, we must acknowledge the fact that these are not constant numbers, as they will vary across patient subgroups.

Inter-rater Reliability

Inter-rater reliability refers to the degree to which the observations of two or more independent raters agree. The outcomes can be expressed using either the intraclass correlation coefficient (ICC) or kappa. Kappa, also known as Cohen's kappa, measures the agreement between two or more raters or observers, particularly for categorical data. A kappa value of 1 indicates perfect agreement. A kappa value of 0 indicates that the agreement is no better than what would be expected by chance. Generally, a kappa score greater than 0.4 indicates moderate agreement, over 0.6 is considered good, and above 0.8 is nearly perfect.

In addition, the ICC is used for continuous data and assesses the reliability of measurements made by different raters. For the ICC, we aim for a score higher than 0.75 to be considered good, with a preference for scores above 0.9 for use in clinical settings. Understanding these differences is crucial for selecting the appropriate measure of agreement based on the type of data being analyzed.

Tissue Irritability

The irritability of your muscles, tendons, ligaments, etc., can best be described as the ability of this tissue to handle physical stress. For example, how do your tendons and muscles respond after you have exercised? Do you experience stiff muscles afterward? Do your tendons become painful? How long does this last, and when did the pain start? All of this determines your tissue irritability.

Why is this important? It is believed that exercise programs are best structured based on your tissue irritability. Generally, three levels of tissue irritability are described:

1. High tissue irritability: You experience significant pain with arm movements in various directions, often rating it above 7/10. Additionally, you frequently feel pain at rest and during the night. When the therapist moves your arm, they are unable to test the full range of motion due to the pain, although they can achieve a greater range compared to when you attempt the movement actively.
2. Moderate tissue irritability: You experience moderate pain with arm movements, typically ranging from 4 to 6/10. You occasionally feel pain at rest and during the night. Your range of motion is nearly the same whether you move your arm yourself or the therapist moves your shoulder.
3. Low tissue irritability: You experience minimal pain with arm movements, typically less than 3/10, and you have no pain at rest or during the night. Your range of motion is consistent whether you move your arm yourself or the therapist moves your shoulder.

Multidimensional Load-Capacity Model

The multidimensional load-capacity model has long been the cornerstone of our clinical reasoning. It aligns well with the biopsychosocial framework, offering a robust approach for developing explanatory models for various conditions. Additionally, its clarity makes it accessible for patients, facilitating effective communication about their complaints.

This model is grounded in a comprehensive load-capacity analysis, where "load" encompasses not only the physical stress on joints but also psychological and social stressors.

Load can be classified as general or local. General load includes broad factors such as prolonged physical exertion, increased work-related stress, alcohol abuse, and infections. Local load, on the other hand, pertains to tissue-specific stress, such as the mechanical strain on the rotator cuff during work or recreational activities. The load is then compared to the patient's capacity to endure it, known as general capacity, or to the tissue's capacity, referred to as local capacity.

Patients may experience reduced general capacity due to factors like decreased fitness, fatigue, poor sleep, age, stress, or increased susceptibility to infections. Similarly, local capacity may be diminished due to previous trauma, anatomical abnormalities, scarring, degeneration, or local inflammatory processes.

Shared Decision-Making

Once the physical examination is complete, ask the patient to take a seat. Express your appreciation for sharing all the information and allowing the examination of their shoulder. Thank them for their cooperation and openness during the process.

Shared decision-making aims to address the asymmetrical relationship between clinicians and patients. This means that as a clinician, you will make a treatment decision together with the patient. This collaborative approach helps the patient engage more easily in the treatment plan afterward. In clinical reasoning, we must be mindful of the patient's knowledge, experiences, and preferences so that these can be incorporated into the decision-making process. You will provide the patient with information about the available treatment options, along with their pros and cons. This initiates the process known as *shared decision-making.*

If the patient asks what you would do, be honest. Give the person the same attention and care you would give to your mother, father, child, best friend, or loved one. Make them feel important and cared for. Take the time to listen and understand them. Communicate with empathy and respect and work together to make decisions through shared decision-making. By doing this, you build a therapeutic relationship with the patient, making them feel safe and understood.

Did the Patient Understand?

To determine whether the patient has understood your explanation, you can start by asking the patient who they will share the information with. Then ask what they will tell them. Based on the patient's response, you can assess if the information has been clearly conveyed. Obviously, if this is not the case, it is up to you as clinician to present the information in a different way.

Finding enough time for this can sometimes be challenging. If that is the case, sending health information via email could be a solution. You can refer the patient to specifically selected informational videos or texts. During a potential follow-up appointment, you can discuss with the patient what they saw in the videos or understood from the texts. When the patient indicates what was difficult to understand, you can focus on educating them about that topic, discuss it, and, if necessary, provide additional resources.

A Schematic Overview of Shoulder Examination

In a schematic overview of the examination, we propose a framework that can provide structure for the assessment of the shoulder (Fig. 8.9). This structure ensures a systematic approach to evaluating symptoms of a stiff, weak, unstable, neurogenic, or inflammatory shoulder.

The process begins with taking a thorough history including screening for serious pathology or other non-musculoskeletal sources of shoulder pain. Next, a comprehensive physical examination is performed, possibly supplemented by specific tests. Additionally, imaging such as X-rays, MRI, or ultrasound may be used to further support the diagnosis.

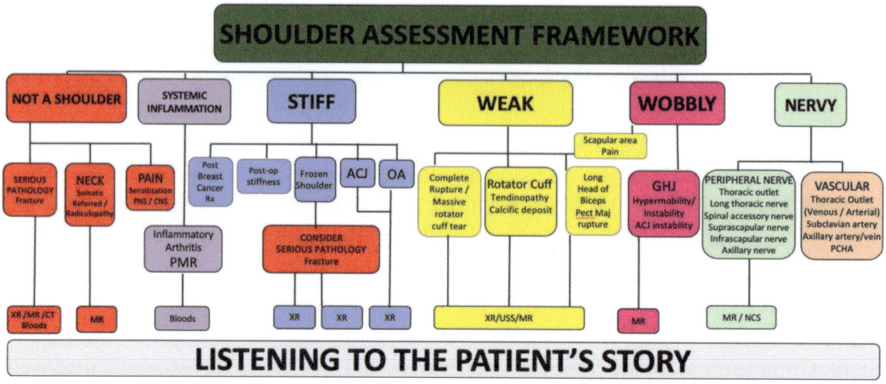

Fig. 8.9 Schematic overview of the clinical examination of the shoulder. Based on personal communication with Eoin Ó Conaire (www.ebtc.ie). Abbreviations: *XR* X-ray, *USS* ultrasound scan, *MR* magnetic resonance imaging, *NCS* nerve conduction study, *CT* computed tomography, *ACJ* acromioclavicular joint, *OA* osteoarthritis, *GHJ* glenohumeral joint, *PCHA* posterior circumflex humeral artery

The framework aims to provide structure in the complexity of a patient with shoulder pain. A more detailed discussion of the various conditions will follow later in this book.

9 Rotator Cuff-Related Shoulder Pain

Let us begin with the most common shoulder condition, previously known as shoulder impingement syndrome, now referred to as rotator cuff-related shoulder pain (RCRSP) [117]. Rotator cuff disorders are the most common cause of shoulder pain, with a lifetime prevalence of approximately 70% [118, 119].

What Is Rotator Cuff-Related Shoulder Pain?

RCRSP was first described in 1972 [120] as impingement of the rotator cuff under the "roof" of the shoulder, namely, the coracoacromial ligament and the anterior third of the acromion. The tendons must pass through a small space between the roof of the shoulder (acromion) and the head of the humerus—known as the subacromial space. It was often suggested that RCRSP is caused by a narrowing of this subacromial space, which would lead to compression of muscles and tendons passing through, leading to degeneration and pain. This was initially described as shoulder impingement syndrome, and since then, many treatments have focused on increasing this space.

However, the cause of RCRSP appears to be more complex and dependent on multiple factors, such as overloading of the rotator cuff, shoulder instability, or possibly a scapular movement disorder. Other causes have also been identified. The varied nature of these potential mechanisms suggests that RCRSP is not a homogeneous entity but rather a heterogeneous syndrome. A lack of understanding regarding the cause often hinders us from initiating successful treatment. A critical review of the impingement concept is essential for gaining insight and selecting the most effective therapeutic option to restore normal shoulder function.

Inherent to this syndrome and its associated therapies is the widespread belief that the aforementioned subacromial space has become too small for the structures passing through it, resulting in compression and pain. But is this really the case? This theory has become quite controversial [121]. The subacromial space is defined by the acromion and coracoacromial ligament as the upper boundary and the

F. Struyf, *Shoulder Pain*, https://doi.org/10.1007/978-3-031-82228-5_9

humeral head as the lower boundary. A reduction in this space can only occur if either the upper boundary moves downward, the lower boundary moves upward, or both simultaneously. The lowering of the upper boundary is described in the scientific literature as either a positional change of the acromion (and thus the scapula), an inappropriate shape of the acromion, or osteophyte formation under the acromion. Let's dive into these options.

A movement disorder of the scapula is called scapular dyskinesis. Scapular dyskinesis is defined as an alteration in the normal movement pattern of the scapula and has been observed in patients with RCRSP [23]. Due to these findings, it is often assumed that shoulder pain develops because of scapular dyskinesis, as these movement disorders could theoretically cause a downward shift of the acromion, thereby reducing the subacromial space. However, it has not been proven that scapular dyskinesis is the cause of shoulder pain.

Several studies have followed overhead athletes, such as in tennis and handball, over long periods to predict shoulder pain based on the presence of scapular dyskinesis. While two studies [122, 123] show a significant predictive value of scapular dyskinesis, four other studies [124–127] do not. Notably, the predictive value reported in [122] was corrected by a later study [127], which added an equivalent number of female athletes to the sample, while the findings in [123] are confounded by the inclusion of cases with traumatic onset of pain, where scapular dyskinesis is unlikely to be the primary cause.

It is clear that the scapula plays a crucial role in the proper functioning of the shoulder. However, various studies have contributed to the cause-and-effect debate regarding the scapula. It has been proven that muscle activity in patients with shoulder pain can change because of the pain [128–130]. These changes in muscle activity, in turn, cause a movement disorder of the scapula, making it clear that this is often a consequence of the pain and not necessarily the cause of any impingement.

This brings us to another possible cause of the reduction in the subacromial space: the shape of the acromion. It has been previously suggested that the shape of the acromion contributes to the narrowing of the subacromial space. Various acromion shapes have been described, such as the flat, hooked, and curved type. Based on the mechanistic theory of impingement, it has been proposed that the hooked type could be a possible cause of impingement. The angle of the acromion can potentially irritate the rotator cuff and cause symptoms. However, strong evidence supporting this is currently lacking [131, 132].

Consequently, it is not surprising that after analyzing 140 patients with shoulder impingement symptoms using MRI—some who underwent subacromial decompression and others who did not—no significant differences were found between the two groups in terms of the number of rotator cuff tears or changes in rotator cuff muscle volume after 5 years [133]. This was confirmed a few years later in a large-scale arthroscopic study with three groups (all RCRSP): arthroscopic subacromial decompression, arthroscopy without intervention, and no intervention. The results showed that increasing the subacromial space offered no added value compared to arthroscopy without intervention and no clinical advantage compared to a control group without surgery [134]. These findings were later reinforced by a systematic review with meta-analysis, which concluded that subacromial decompression as a standard intervention is not justified as a treatment for RCRSP [135].

Does the subacromial space actually have any relationship to shoulder pain? Very little, according to an ultrasound study, which showed no differences between patients with and without impingement symptoms in terms of the size of the subacromial space [136]. Similarly, the percentage of tendon thickness relative to the subacromial space, referred to as the *occupation* ratio, is no different in RCRSP patients compared to healthy individuals. Therefore, the subacromial space likely plays only a minor, often negligible, role in the patient's pain. However, research typically focuses on the "average patient," and as we all know, that average patient is rarely the one who walks into your clinic. In other words, be cautious with terms like "never" and "always." The subacromial space may still play a relevant role in a specifically selected group of patients.

Moreover, the term "impingement" might be a misrepresentation [137, 138] and can have a nocebo effect. The word suggests a mechanical issue that can lead to avoidance behaviors. I might think that if I move my shoulder, my tendons will get pinched and the pain will worsen and therefore avoid those movements. Makes sense, right? But by doing so, the muscles and tendons around the shoulder are used even less, losing much of their strength, quality, and thus capacity to resist load. This, in turn, will cause problems the next time the patient performs a household task. Accurately diagnosing a condition can make treatment more effective, but that is not always the case with anatomically based diagnoses like "impingement."

Fortunately, recent international literature offers new opportunities. These opportunities lie in creating a patient profile based on all aspects of the *International Classification of Functioning* (ICF). From this perspective, it appears that several factors are linked to RCRSP [137]. First, there is an imbalance between the demands placed on the rotator cuff and its ability to meet them. This is referred to as an imbalance between the load and capacity of the rotator cuff. It is a mechanism at the root of many tendon problems, including in shoulder patients with RCRSP. Indeed, RCRSP largely refers to a tendon problem—tendinopathy—of the rotator cuff.

But it goes beyond that. In fact, it turns out that alcohol use, hormones, genetics, smoking, diabetes, and psychosocial factors can all influence the development and persistence of RCRSP. All these factors can create a situation where even a small or significant overload can lead to symptoms—a perfect environment for an inflammatory response. In any case, it is clear that our shoulder tendons were not prepared for a particular task. But how exactly do these factors influence the tendon structure and its ability to handle load? To understand this, we need to take a closer look at the composition and function of our tendons.

Our tendons consist of multiple layers and are primarily made up of water, collagen, and a small amount of elastin. Rotator cuff tendon tissue is about 70% water, with the rest (mainly) being type I collagen bound by the interfascicular matrix. The latter provides structure to the tendon. Type I collagen (typically produced by fibroblasts) forms tendon units, which are fascicles of fiber bundles. The fiber bundles, in turn, are composed of fibrils, all aligned parallel to the long axis of the tendon. Thick and strong muscles create thick and strong tendons. The force of a muscle must be transferred to the bone to create movement. As a muscle gets stronger, so does the tendon, to fulfill its part of the task. Our tendons must work hard daily. In addition to frictional and compressive forces, they primarily endure tensile forces: the muscle pulls on the tendon. It is clear that tendons are essential for movement in our bodies, and they must be strong enough to withstand these tensile forces. A tendon must adapt by becoming stronger when the muscle pulls on it frequently and powerfully but weaker when the muscle pulls on it infrequently or lightly. The tendon adapts like a true chameleon.

Various cells play a role in the creation and maintenance of tendons, such as tenocytes, tenoblasts, fibroblasts, chondrocytes, and so on. Tenoblasts are immature cells that later develop into tenocytes. The latter help maintain a balance between the breakdown and buildup of our tendons. When do tenocytes become active? Precisely when they detect tensile forces in the tendon. These tensile forces—a type of mechanical stimulus—trigger intracellular processes that enhance collagen synthesis. However, tensile forces also cause some breakdown, likely as an initial response to the load, followed by the tenocytes' reaction to strengthen the tissue again. By allowing the tendon to rest after an exercise session, the buildup will surpass the breakdown, and the tendon will become stronger.

If there is an imbalance between the buildup and breakdown of tendon tissue, the term "tendinopathy" emerges. Tendinopathy is considered the preferred term for persistent tendon pain and loss of function related to mechanical load. The tendon will weaken. It is still unclear whether a degenerative tendon can fully heal. However, this does not mean that improvement cannot occur. Even in a degenerative tendon, there are healthy areas that have the potential to regain strength. This concept is illustrated by the "donut theory." In this analogy, the tendon is compared to a donut, where the hole symbolizes the tendon issue. The idea is to focus on treating the donut—the healthy sections of the tendon—rather than the hole.

The effect of load on a tendon can also vary depending on intrinsic risk factors such as genetics, obesity, age, and loading history. We also cannot ignore the substantial evidence of inflammation in and around the tendon. In the past, the term "tendinitis" was abandoned due to the belief that there was no real inflammation. However, the evidence for inflammation is quite clear. Pro-inflammatory cells are significantly increased in the rotator cuff tendons in cases of tendinopathy. Tendon disorders are highly complex. Even with the vast amount of research published on this topic, it remains difficult to fully understand the inflammatory response.

If the evidence for impingement of subacromial structures is lacking, and we have increasing evidence of an intrinsic or tendinous origin of the pain, we should be able to provide the patient with a clear, understandable, and above all "correct" explanation of their pain. This explanation might include "Your pain is likely coming from the muscles and tendons in and around your shoulder. These muscles and tendons have insufficient capacity, which may be the reason for the pain you feel when lifting your arm. This capacity, for example, refers to tendon strength. Due to this lack of capacity, your tendons and muscles become overloaded, resulting in pain."

How Do you Recognize Rotator Cuff-Related Shoulder Pain?

Patients aged 50 or older, those with diabetes, and individuals who frequently perform overhead activities are at the highest risk for rotator cuff tendinopathy [139]. The clinical presentation typically includes vague pain around the shoulder when lifting the arm, sometimes radiating to the upper arm and elbow. Other shoulder conditions such as frozen shoulder, glenohumeral instability, neck pain, or pain from trauma should be ruled out (Table 9.1).

Step 1: Rule Out a Frozen Shoulder

A frozen shoulder (FS) is a pathology characterized by the spontaneous onset of shoulder pain accompanied by gradual limitations in both active and passive shoulder movements [140]. Diagnosing FS can be challenging and is sometimes initially confused with various differential diagnoses, such as (osteo)arthritis (OA), posterior dislocation, subacromial shoulder pain, and postoperative shoulder stiffness [141, 142]. For a diagnosis of FS, the ROM must be restricted by at least 25% in at least two planes of movement and more than 50% in external rotation (with the arm in 0 degrees of abduction) compared to the unaffected side. The symptoms must also be stable or worsening for at least 1 month [143]. Have a look at the chapter on frozen shoulder for a more detailed discussion of this condition and its clinical presentation.

Table 9.1 Clinical presentation of rotator cuff-related shoulder pain

Inclusion criteria	Exclusion criteria
Pain in the deltoid region and upper arm	
Pain during shoulder movements	Previous trauma (e.g., subluxation, dislocation; except for microinstability)
Preexisting pain when reaching overhead or bringing the hand behind the back	Pain at rest
Pain when lying on the shoulder is possible	
	Pain triggered by neck movements
	Distal neurovascular symptoms
	Significant loss of ROM
	Severe loss of external rotation ROM
	Decrease in external rotation ROM with increased abduction
Typical pain present with loading, in particular, in shoulder abduction and external rotation	

Step 2: Rule Out Shoulder Pain of Cervical Origin

In an international Delphi study, physical therapists specializing in shoulder care have come to an agreement on important factors to consider when screening the spine in individuals with shoulder pain. These factors include the location of symptoms distal to the shoulder, any current or past neck pain, symptom changes associated with neck movements, and the presence of neuropathic-like symptoms. Although it is usually sufficient to examine the neck in patients presenting with shoulder pain through an active range of motion test of the neck to see if it provokes any shoulder pain, this Delphi study also highlighted the significance of adding the Spurling test and techniques for modifying symptoms related to the spine [144]. We refer to the chapter on neurological-related shoulder problems and more specifically the cervical radiculopathy section, for further reading.

Step 3: Rule Out Trauma-Related Pain

Ruling out trauma-related pain is primarily based on history taking. If the patient reports such trauma, imaging may be used to rule out a shoulder fracture or dislocation. On the other hand, glenohumeral instability may also be present. Shoulder instability often begins with a specific incident or activity, indicating a possible structural lesion. Both anterior and posterior instability can also involve one or more incidents of dislocation or subluxation.

However, international Delphi shoulder experts reached a consensus that rotator cuff tears in younger patients (under 40) can stem from either traumatic or atraumatic causes, particularly in the context of overhead sports, where microinstability may develop. However, the relationship between microinstability and rotator cuff disorders is debated, with some suggesting that this laxity might even serve as a protective mechanism against impingement [145].

Anterior instability is typically characterized by a positive *apprehension, relocation, and release test,* where the patient reports typical symptoms such as a feeling of instability, fear of movement, and clicking when the arm is placed in abduction and external rotation. We will discuss this further in the chapter on glenohumeral instability.

Step 4: Eliciting the Typical Pain in RCRSP

Would you like to perform additional tests to support your diagnosis? There are dozens of tests available, but they come with various challenges. Strong systematic reviews and even meta-analyses have investigated the sensitivity, specificity, and *likelihood* ratios of different orthopedic tests for shoulder pain [146, 147]. The results, however, are disappointing. Aside from standardizing the reproduction of pain, these tests do not offer much extra information. Even when combining different orthopedic tests, there was only a limited increase in clinimetric accuracy [147]. This could be for several reasons. First, all clinical tests are positive based on the symptom of pain, which is a very subjective and unreliable indicator in patients with chronic pain syndromes. Second, imaging techniques like ultrasound, MRI, or arthroscopy are often used as the reference standard to assess the accuracy of clinical tests [148]. However, this method is highly questioned, especially given the weak relationship between imaging findings and patient symptoms [136, 149–157]. Third, the lack of reliable diagnostic tests for RCRSP can be explained by changes in the mechanosensitivity of the soft tissues in the shoulder [158]. This means that any cause of shoulder inflammation can lead to an irritable shoulder joint, making it difficult to distinguish between different shoulder conditions or anatomical structures. A Delphi study among international shoulder experts also reported that no items reached consensus within the "special tests" diagnostic domain [145]. Finally, the validity of these tests can also be questioned, as they primarily aim to reduce the subacromial space to provoke pain. However, if the subacromial space is not the main cause of shoulder pain, these tests are essentially targeting a mechanism that may not be relevant.

Pain related to mechanical load is a key indicator of rotator cuff-related shoulder pain (RCRSP) in subjective assessments. While RCRSP has multiple causes, poor load management—such as excessive or altered loading on subacromial structures—appears to be a primary factor influencing its development and progression. Pain behavior in RCRSP resembles that of tendinopathies, showing variability based on load. This condition is particularly common among active individuals and those involved in overhead sports, often affecting the dominant shoulder. The Delphi study experts noted that pain is the most frequently reported in the deltoid region, with some cases extending to the forearm [145].

Due to the limited clinical value of these additional tests and the uncertainty of imaging in confirming a diagnosis or determining which tissues are responsible for the patient's symptoms, our clinical reasoning has shifted toward identifying treatable factors. One such method is the use of symptom modification procedures [159–161]. This includes techniques like manually correcting the scapula during arm movements. If symptoms improve, the complaint may be attributed to the scapula, giving us a treatable factor. For instance, there is the *scapular retraction test* (SRT), where you ask the patient to place their arms in the *empty can* position while the clinician stabilizes the scapula of the affected side in a posterior tilt and external rotation. You then apply downward pressure on the affected arm (as in the *empty can test*) and assess whether scapular retraction reduces symptoms. Symptom reduction is considered a positive test, possibly indicating scapular involvement? Unfortunately, it is not that simple. Further research of this method sometimes led to surprising results. A positive SRT was found to be related to the status of the rotator cuff [162]. Surprising but not irrational. Many scapular symptom modification tests seem to assist the rotator cuff in its function. Symptom reduction could therefore provide information about both the rotator cuff and the scapula.

Two things are certain: first, a positive symptom modification test likely points to a musculoskeletal problem, which is why these tests are often positive in rotator cuff-related issues. However, this approach clearly requires further research. Second, our special clinical tests are not as special as we once thought when it comes to diagnosing RCRSP [163]. As previously mentioned, there is a clear lack of diagnostic accuracy in the special orthopedic tests commonly used for RCRSP. Recognizable pain should be reproduced with load/resistance tests, which typically involve abduction with external rotation. For this reason, provocative tests are valuable in standardizing the typical pain pattern in your patients.

Biceps Tendon Pathology

10

Some researchers consider the musculus biceps brachii (m. biceps brachii) and its long head (*long head biceps tendon*, LHBT) as part of the pathological picture in rotator cuff-related shoulder pain. Therefore, they recommend a clinical examination and a treatment plan aligned with RCRSP. While we certainly understand this approach, we have dedicated a separate chapter to this specific pathology due to the fundamental differences in anatomy, biomechanics, function, and management.

It is indeed often observed that there is concurrent rotator cuff pathology present with LHBT tendinopathy. Notably, there are strong associations with the tendon of the subscapularis muscle (m. subscapularis). Additionally, isolated tears of the supraspinatus muscle (m. supraspinatus) and m. subscapularis have been found in combination with LHBT instability. For example, it is also common to see rotator cuff tears in the absence of the LHBT.

The long head of the biceps brachii muscle originates from the supraglenoid tubercle and the superior labrum, passing through the rotator cuff interval. This tendon runs intra-articular until it exits the glenohumeral capsule and continues through the intertubercular groove. Further down, the LHBT merges with the short head to form the m. biceps brachii.

Distally, there is only one tendon, which attaches at the level of the radius. The literature describes several anatomical variations in the m. biceps brachii, both proximally and distally, with frequent reports of a congenitally absent LHBT. Much has been written and debated about the anatomy and especially the function of the m. biceps brachii and the LHBT [164]. Aside from the logical activity of the m. biceps brachii during elbow flexion, supination, and some shoulder anteflexion, there is also consensus that, in healthy shoulders, the LHBT plays a role in shoulder movements from 90 degrees of abduction, typically during overhead arm movements.

Multiple studies indicate that the m. biceps brachii plays a stabilizing role in the glenohumeral joint. However, there is limited direct evidence regarding the involvement of the long head of the biceps tendon (LHBT) in shoulder proprioception. Conversely, shoulder pain may influence how the biceps brachii is recruited. Could it be the other way around?

F. Struyf, *Shoulder Pain*, https://doi.org/10.1007/978-3-031-82228-5_10

Unfortunately, the functional role of the LHBT in the shoulder is still not well understood, and its contribution to shoulder movement and stability remains unclear. In addition, the impact of LHBT surgery on shoulder function and the progression of rotator cuff pathology remains unknown.

What Are the LHBT Pathologies?

The most common pathologies associated with the LHBT are tendon instability, tendinopathy, tendon ruptures, and superior labrum anterior-posterior (SLAP) lesions. The latter will be discussed in a separate chapter.

Instability of the LHBT is a common cause of shoulder pain. We clearly see that the LHBT must make a sharp turn when it exits the intertubercular groove. The capsuloligamentous sling, consisting of the superior glenohumeral ligament (SGHL) and the coracohumeral ligament (CHL), plays a stabilizing and supportive role in this sharp bend as the LHBT moves from the intertubercular groove to the supraglenoid tuberosity. The superior insertion of the subscapularis tendon also plays a crucial role in maintaining the integrity of the LHBT. All of this prevents anteromedial displacement of the LHBT.

The first signs of biceps instability can be subtle, with only a slight medial displacement of the LHBT. Severe subluxations or dislocations of the LHBT from the bicipital groove can be easily identified through imaging. Various researchers have developed different classification systems. The simplest describe only three patterns based on the direction of the luxation to medial, lateral or both [165].

The LHBT is of particular interest due to its association with the rotator cuff, where tendinopathy can occur from repetitive shoulder motions. Pain at the LHBT is no different from other tendon pain, being a complex, multifaceted experience initiated by noxious stimuli, involving sensory and emotional components influenced by social and environmental factors [166]. Chronic LHBT pain, particularly associated with tendinopathy, remains poorly understood. LHBT tendinopathy refers to tendon pathology characterized by the disruption of normal collagen structure, often linked to overuse, resulting in pain during activity and reduced functional strength.

How Do You Recognize an LHBT Pathology?

As with RCRSP, we are dealing with limited diagnostic value from individual orthopedic tests. Several systematic reviews and diagnostic studies have examined the validity of orthopedic tests for LHBT pathology and have shown substantial variability. This variability can partly be explained by the different presentations of LHBT patients: reactive tendinopathy versus degenerative tendinopathy. In any case, the clinical picture often resembles that of RCRSP patients and frequently that of patients with labrum lesions as well.

The patient will almost always report symptoms at the anterior side of the shoulder. During the reactive phase, the symptoms can be quite intense at night, especially when the patient lies on the affected side, and the pain is often rather sharp. In the more chronic phase, the pain becomes more blunted and is described as dull. During both the reactive and degenerative phases, symptoms can radiate along the anterior/lateral side of the upper arm.

Tests such as the Yergason test (LR+ 1.94 and LR− 0.74) (Fig. 10.1) and the uppercut maneuver (LR+ 3.38 and LR− 0.34) (Fig. 10.2) could potentially be valuable [167–170]. The Yergason test is particularly useful when the result is positive, while the uppercut maneuver is informative for both negative and positive results. Unfortunately, the clinimetric properties of these tests are not outstanding, resulting in only a slight increase or decrease in the likelihood of LHBT pathology. Combining these orthopedic tests does little to enhance their effectiveness [147, 171].

The Yergason Test

During the Yergason test (see Fig. 10.1), the patient sits or stands while you, the practitioner, stand beside the patient on the affected side. Ask the patient to flex the elbow at 90 degrees and pronate the forearm. With your opposite hand, palpate

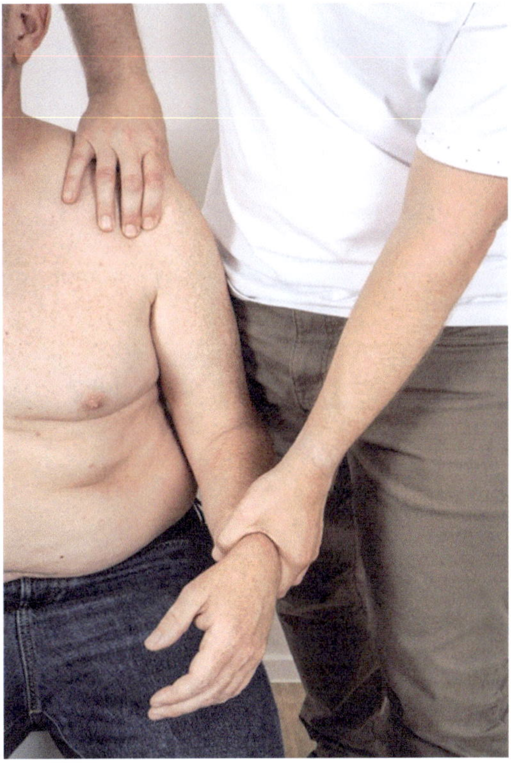

Fig. 10.1 The Yergason test

the long head of the biceps tendon in the intertubercular sulcus. Grasp the patient's wrist with your corresponding hand. Ask the patient to simultaneously flex the elbow and supinate the forearm. You apply resistance to both movements.

The test is positive if the patient feels pain around the bicipital groove and/or if there is subluxation of the long head of the biceps.

The Uppercut Maneuver

During the uppercut maneuver (Fig. 10.2a, b), the patient sits or stands while you, the practitioner, stand beside them on the affected side. You then ask the patient to actively lift their arm and bring it into slight internal rotation, with the elbow flexed, as if performing an uppercut, while you apply resistance throughout the entire movement.

The test is positive if the patient experiences pain around the bicipital groove and/or if there is subluxation of the long head of the biceps.

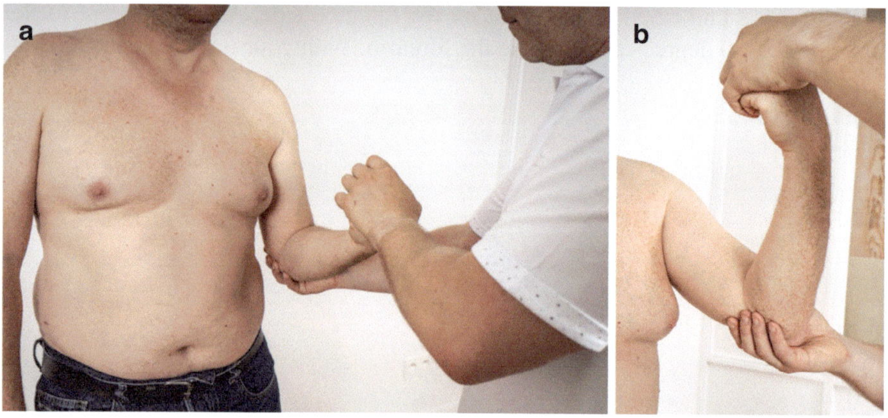

Fig. 10.2 (**a, b**) The uppercut maneuver

11 Labral Injury

The glenoid labrum consists of a fibrous, cartilaginous, oval-shaped structure. For the most part, the labrum adheres closely to the edge of the glenoid. The long head of the biceps brachii muscle attaches to the supraglenoid tubercle and the superior part of the labrum. However, numerous anatomical variations have been described [172].

Under normal conditions, the labrum is well rounded and mobile in relation to the glenoid, but in some cases, part of the labrum may become detached or even be absent. The labrum serves as a passive stabilizer to prevent subluxation of the humeral head [173, 174].

What Is a Labral Injury?

Labral injuries are often linked to issues with the long head biceps tendon (LHBT). This connection is due not only to their shared anatomical region but also because they frequently occur in the same population. In 1990, the term SLAP lesion was introduced [175], which stands for superior labrum, anterior to posterior.

Labral injuries are typically classified by their location. For example, Snyder described six labral regions (Fig. 11.1) [175].

In a stable shoulder, labral injuries primarily occur in sector 1, where the long head of the biceps brachii muscle attaches. Sectors 4 and 5 are rare here [176].

The main mechanisms causing labral injuries include compression trauma from the humeral head against the labrum [177], heavy lifting [178, 179] repetitive overhead movements, traction trauma, or microtrauma due to a *peel-back* mechanism [175, 180, 181].

Isolated SLAP lesions are rare, and many patients have additional injuries, such as rotator cuff tears or instability [182]. However, having a SLAP lesion does not necessarily mean there is pain. These injuries are often documented in a large number of asymptomatic individuals [183, 184].

F. Struyf, *Shoulder Pain*, https://doi.org/10.1007/978-3-031-82228-5_11

Fig. 11.1 Labral locations based on Snyder's classification [175]

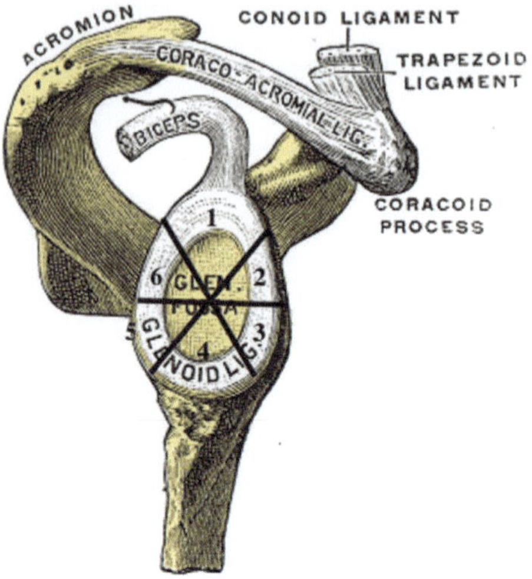

Labral Tears in Sector 1 (SLAP Lesions)

SLAP stands for superior labrum from anterior to posterior, although the location of these lesions typically runs from posterior to anterior. These injuries occur in the complex involving the labrum and the long head of the biceps brachii muscle, corresponding to sector 1 according to Snyder. It is estimated that the majority (80–90%) of labral injuries are SLAP lesions, though they are only visible in about 6% of shoulder arthroscopies [185]. As mentioned earlier, anatomical variants can sometimes present a similar appearance, making interpretation challenging. SLAP lesions can be categorized into eight types, ranging from degenerative lesions to various types of labral tears depending on their shape and size.

Labral Tears in Sector 2 and Sector 6

Sector 2 labral tears involve the anterior labrum and are often accompanied by a tear of the medial glenohumeral ligament.

Sector 6 labral tears are located posteriorly and are less common than sector 1 and 2 labral tears. This type of labral tear can extend superiorly to a SLAP lesion and is frequently seen in overhead throwers due to the peel-back phenomenon in an abduction external rotation position of the shoulder [186]. The pain is often explained by impingement of the posterior labrum.

Labral Tears in Sector 3 and Sector 4

These tears are located in the anterior and inferior regions and are often associated with anterior shoulder instability. Additionally, tears of the inferior and/or medial glenohumeral ligament are commonly seen, with or without accompanying bone injuries in the same area. A *gleno-labral articular disruption* (GLAD) lesion can sometimes be observed here. This involves an impact injury on the anterior edge of the glenoid.

Bankart lesions are also found in these anterior and inferior sectors. They involve a detachment of the anterior labrum, which may or may not be associated with an accompanying anterior bone injury. A Bankart lesion can sometimes extend superiorly and reach a SLAP lesion.

Labral Tears in Sector 5

Posterior and inferior labral tears are typically associated with posterior instability, which occurs much less frequently than anterior instability. These lesions are sometimes referred to as reverse Bankart lesions. As with anterior tears, they may also be accompanied by cartilage damage.

How Do You Recognize a Labral Injury

The clinical presentation of a patient with a labral injury can be highly variable, making SLAP lesions difficult to diagnose. They often occur alongside other shoulder pathologies, and the reported diagnostic accuracy of examination tests is generally poor. Some patients may report a clicking or locking sensation, while others feel as though something shifts in the shoulder. Symptoms can range from instability to stiffness, but the most common complaints are usually pain or instability. Also, a feeling of weakness when the arm is in 90 degrees of abduction and external rotation is common.

The clinical assessment of labral injuries is based on the patient's history, physical examination, and imaging. There are some specific clinical tests that are considered reliable for detecting labral injuries [187]. However, they are often not sensitive or specific enough to definitively diagnose a SLAP lesion [167, 188]. More recent research suggests that a combination of two tests, the biceps load I (+LR: 29.09; –LR: 0.09) and biceps load II (+LR: 26.32; –LR: 0.11) [187], may be sufficient to diagnose a SLAP lesion [189].

The Biceps Load I Test

The test is performed in supine. You, the practitioner, stand beside the patient and hold their elbow and wrist. Bring the arm into 90 degrees of abduction and 90 degrees of elbow flexion, with the forearm in supination. Ask the patient to relax. Next, move the arm into maximum external rotation while keeping the upper arm in 90 degrees of abduction. Then instruct the patient to bend their elbow.

This test is positive if the typical pain occurs (Fig. 11.2).

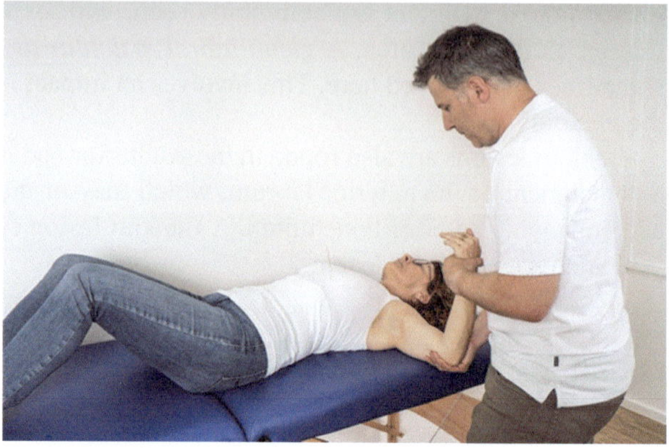

Fig. 11.2 The biceps load I test

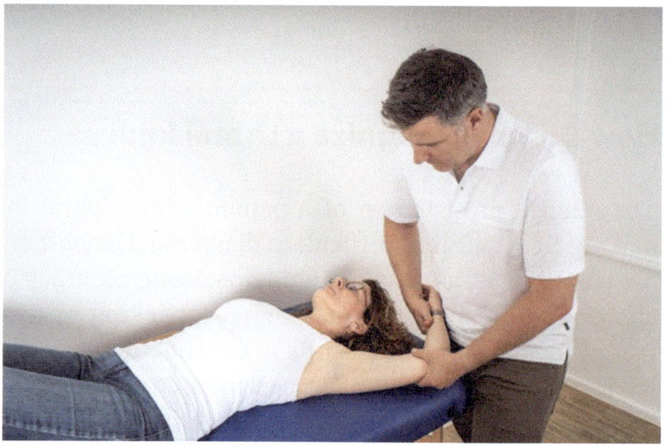

Fig. 11.3 The biceps load II test

The Biceps Load II Test

The test is also performed in supine. You, the practitioner, stand next to the patient and hold the elbow and wrist. Position the shoulder in 120 degrees of abduction and maximum external rotation, with the elbow at 90 degrees of flexion and the forearm in supination. Ask the patient to flex their elbow while you apply resistance.

This test is considered positive if pain occurs during resisted elbow flexion or if there is more pain when resisting elbow flexion than before (Fig. 11.3).

Rotator Cuff Tears 12

Rotator cuff tears are quite common, but there is currently little consensus on whether these structural changes in the rotator cuff are actually the cause of shoulder pain. This is because many people with structural changes in their rotator cuff experience no pain [190]. For example, more than 50% of people over 80 have an asymptomatic rotator cuff tear.

Although rotator cuff degeneration increases rapidly in the general population from the age of 50–55 and peaks at 80, most shoulder pain is reported between the ages of 60 and 65. This suggests that there is no proportional relationship between the severity of degeneration and shoulder pain.

What Is a Rotator Cuff Tear?

Rotator cuff tears can be divided into traumatic and nontraumatic tears. Traumatic tears tend to occur more often in younger athletes, while nontraumatic tears are more common in patients over 40. Nontraumatic tears are also referred to as degenerative tears.

But which tears cause the most pain? And does the amount of shoulder pain give us an idea of the size of the tear? Not really. First of all, pain is a poor indicator of the size of the tear. In fact, small partial tears can cause more pain than a fully torn tendon [191]. More importantly, the location of the tear matters. Tears in the rotator cable, the thick fibrous bundle that acts like a "suspension bridge" to transmit forces to the rotator cuff, tend to cause more discomfort than tears elsewhere in the rotator cuff.

A specific subgroup of rotator cuff tears is known as massive rotator cuff tears. These are classified as massive when more than one tendon of the rotator cuff is torn [192]. Massive rotator cuff tears make up approximately 10–40% of all rotator cuff tears and 80% of all recurrent tears [193]. Most patients with massive tears are often unable to lift their hand above their head or actively raise the affected arm above shoulder height, a condition referred to as pseudoparalysis [194, 195].

F. Struyf, *Shoulder Pain*, https://doi.org/10.1007/978-3-031-82228-5_12

This occurs mainly when the patient has torn more than one rotator cuff tendon, often involving the entire posterior row of the rotator cuff. As a result, the patient loses control of the humerus in the glenoid cavity, causing the humerus to migrate superiorly and encounter the acromion. This impairs the ability to lift the shoulder, making it appear as though the patient is paralyzed. However, this is not a neurological issue; the nerve function is still perfectly fine. The problem lies in the rotator cuff's inability to perform its primary function of keeping the humeral head centered in the glenoid. While some of these patients can be asymptomatic, many experience worsening pain and weakness in the involved shoulder and pain when they elevate the affected arm above shoulder height or in some cases above 45 degrees [193].

Not all massive rotator cuff tears are irreparable. However, in elderly patients, the poor quality of tendon tissue can lead to high failure rates in surgical repairs. It is suggested to base clinical decision-making on at least four criteria: degree of tendon retraction, the amount of fatty infiltration, the acromiohumeral distance, and a positive tangent sign [193]. The latter is a sign on MRI, when the supraspinatus muscle does not cross a line drawn through specific anatomical landmarks.

How Do You Recognize a Rotator Cuff Tear?

The presentation of patients with a rotator cuff tear can be very variable. Some patients show severe functional limitations, while others may have no symptoms at all [196]. Patients often experience a gradual or insidious onset of pain, typically worsened by activities such as overhead movements, reaching, lifting, carrying, or pushing.

Patients with symptomatic rotator cuff tears generally report pain, mild restrictions in movement, scapular dyskinesis, and increased activation of surrounding shoulder muscles, despite a loss of shoulder muscle strength [130, 196]. The location of the pain resembles that of a rotator cuff-related issue, typically over the anterolateral shoulder, extending into the upper arm and posteriorly near the deltoid muscle.

Positive *drop* or *lag signs* may also be present. The patient might be able to lift their arm to 180 degrees, but when lowering it, the arm suddenly "drops" with an accelerated movement, known as the *drop sign*. A *lag sign*, on the other hand, indicates the patient's inability to hold the arm in a certain position. However, the clinimetric properties of these tests are not perfect, so they should be used with caution. In cases of massive tears, patients may exhibit pseudoparalysis.

Usually, a cluster of clinical tests is recommended [147, 196], such as a combination of the *drop sign* [197] (sensitivity 73%, specificity 77%) and an *external rotation lag sign* (sensitivity 97%, specificity 93%) [198] or internal rotation lag sign (sensitivity 100%, specificity 84%) [197]. Additionally, the combination with age >65 years and nocturnal pain increases the likelihood. Weakness in external rotation can be detected with the *external rotation lag sign* [199]. A positive *hornblowers* sign may indicate degeneration of the teres minor muscle (sensitivity

17–100%, specificity 93–96%; LR+4.25) [200, 201]. However, a negative test does not rule out the presence of a tear.

The Drop-Arm Sign

In the *drop-arm sign* (Fig. 12.1a, b), the patient is either seated on the examination table or standing. You, the practitioner, stand on the affected side. Bring the patient's arm into 90 degrees of abduction and some external rotation (forearm can be pronated as in Fig. 12.1). Then ask the patient to hold this position while you remove the support.

This test is positive if the patient is unable to maintain this position and cannot lower the arm slowly and in a controlled manner.

The External Rotation Lag Sign

In the *external rotation lag sign* (Fig. 12.2a, b), the patient is either seated on the examination table or standing. You, the practitioner, position the patient's arm in 90 degrees of abduction and maximal external rotation, with the elbow at 90 degrees

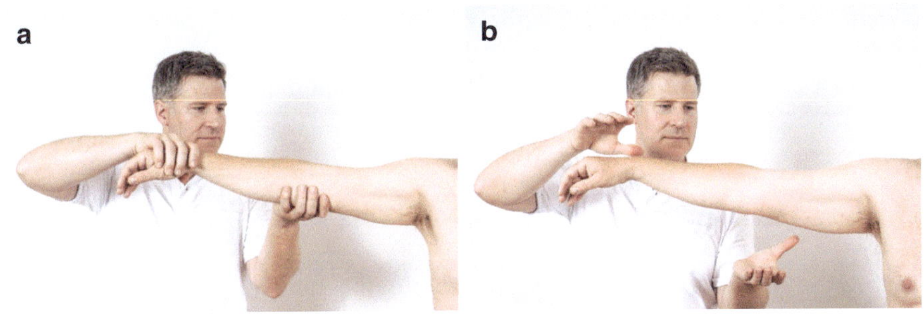

Fig. 12.1 (**a, b**) The drop-arm sign

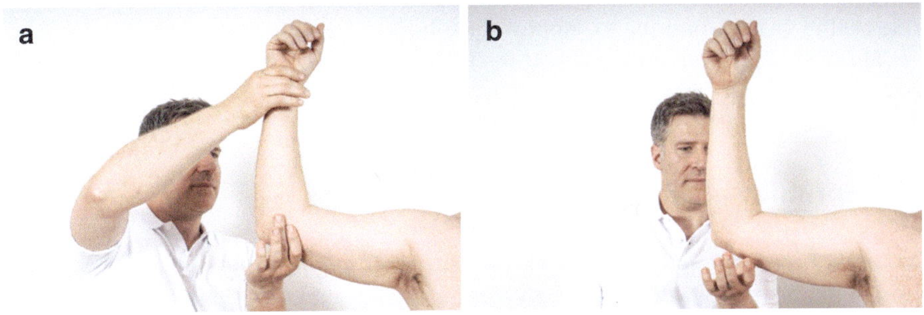

Fig. 12.2 (**a, b**) The external rotation lag sign

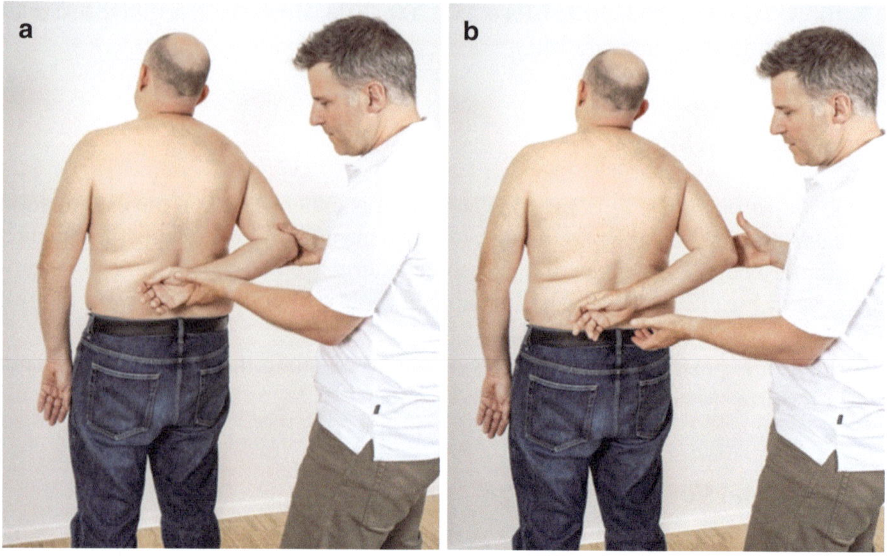

Fig. 12.3 (**a, b**) The *internal rotation lag-sign/lift off test*

of flexion. Then slightly move the shoulder back to avoid elastic recoil. Ask the patient to maintain this position while you release their wrist. The elbow remains supported.

This test is positive if the shoulder moves into internal rotation after releasing the wrist.

The Internal Rotation Lag Sign/Lift-Off Test

In the *internal rotation lag sign* (Fig. 12.3a, b), the patient is either seated on the examination table or standing. The shoulder is internally rotated by bringing the patient's arm behind their back. The elbow is flexed to 90 degrees. The practitioner slightly lifts the shoulder away from the patient's back via the elbow and wrist, stopping just before maximal internal rotation. Ask the patient to hold this position and release the wrist. Continue to support the elbow.

This test is positive if the back of the hand falls against the back once the wrist is released.

The Hornblowers Test

In the *hornblowers test* (Fig. 12.4), the patient sits upright in a chair. The patient brings the arm to 90 degrees of abduction in the scapular plane, with the elbow flexed at 90 degrees. Move the arm into submaximal external rotation and

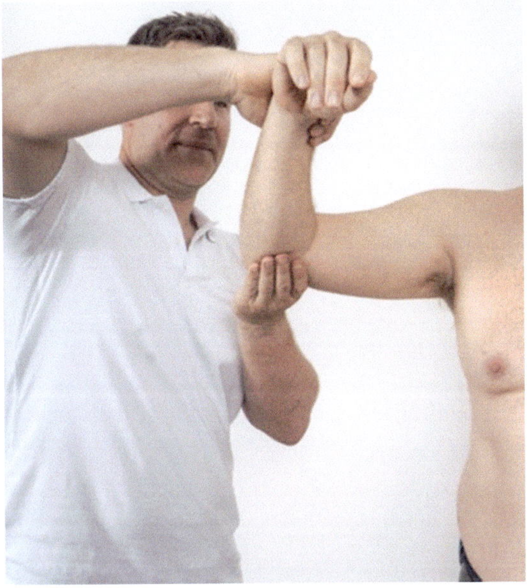

Fig. 12.4 The hornblowers test

ask the patient to externally rotate the forearm against the resistance of the practitioner's hand.

The test is positive if the patient is unable to externally rotate the arm.

Alternative: The same can be assessed by having the patient actively bring their hand toward their mouth. If there is insufficient strength for external rotation, the elbow will be raised during this motion.

13 Calcific Rotator Cuff Tendinopathy

When we think of rotator cuff-related shoulder pain, we automatically think of calcific tendon issues.

Calcific tendinopathy frequently occurs in the tendons of the supraspinatus (80%), infraspinatus (15%), and subscapularis (5%) [202, 203]. It is typically observed in adults between the ages of 30 and 60 [204], and X-rays show its presence in 2.7–10.3% of all adults, while ultrasound and MRI studies report even higher rates, around 20% [202, 205]. Women are slightly more at risk for this condition, as well as patients with hypothyroidism and diabetes.

What Is Calcific Rotator Cuff Tendinopathy?

In the past, various terms have been used, such as calcific tendinitis, calcific periarthritis, and tendinosis calcarea. The term "calcific tendinopathy" is now considered the most appropriate.

Calcium deposits are often detected in people without shoulder pain, but when they cause symptoms, the condition is diagnosed as calcific rotator cuff tendinopathy. Approximately 30–50% of calcified rotator cuff tendons are symptomatic. However, the origin of the calcification remains a mystery. Several hypotheses have been suggested, going from metabolic changes, mechanical overload to age-related changes, and genetic factors. These theories exist, but none have been fully proven. One theory holds steady: under normal conditions, tendon stem cells differentiate into tenocytes, allowing for tendon regeneration and repair. However, under altered conditions, tendon stem cells differentiate into chondrocytes and osteoblasts instead of tenocytes, leading to the formation of calcium deposits within the tendon [206]. The future will tell which theory is dominant or whether it is a combination of different theories.

F. Struyf, *Shoulder Pain*, https://doi.org/10.1007/978-3-031-82228-5_13

The condition has three stages, i.e., precalcification, calcification, and postcalcification, with symptoms reportedly peaking during the calcium resorption process at the end of the calcification stage. The precalcification stage is considered asymptomatic and is characterized by the presence of chondrocyte-like cells.

The calcification stage is divided into a formation phase, resting phase, and resorption phase and can last from several months to several years. During these phases, calcium deposits form and may spontaneously resorb at the end. It is often during this final phase that pain is commonly reported.

The postcalcification stage is no longer painful and involves the remodeling of the tendon tissue. The calcification process can also trigger an inflammatory mechanism. This induces neovascularization and neo-innervation, likely responsible for the pain sensations and observations during power Doppler ultrasound. A positive power Doppler signal within the calcification is indeed strongly associated with pain [207].

How Do You Recognize Calcific Rotator Cuff Tendinopathy?

It may not surprise you to hear that there are currently no specific shoulder tests recommended for diagnosing calcific rotator cuff tendinopathy. Diagnosis involves a thorough medical history and clinical examination, followed by imaging to confirm the presence of calcifications in the rotator cuff tendons. The uncertain relationship between the presence of calcifications and symptoms makes diagnosis challenging. How confident are we that the two are related? It turns out to be about 50/50. At least 50% of rotator cuff calcifications are likely asymptomatic.

Clinically, we already know that most pain occurs during the resorptive phase. This pain can be short lived or last for several weeks [207, 208]. Additionally, patients often report tenderness at the rotator cuff insertion, night pain, and limited range of motion [209]. The pain is less likely to radiate distally compared to RCRSP [210].

14 Frozen Shoulder

A frozen shoulder is also known as adhesive capsulitis. The term "frozen shoulder" is preferred because it covers the entire progression of the condition. Adhesive capsulitis specifically refers to an inflammatory process present only in the early stages of a frozen shoulder.

A frozen shoulder appears to be unique to the shoulder. Although cases of adhesive capsulitis have been reported in the knee, hip, and ankle [211, 212], these are rare exceptions.

What Is a Frozen Shoulder?

While no definite cause has been identified, several key mechanisms are involved in the pathogenesis of a frozen shoulder. The primary cell type within the glenohumeral capsule is the fibroblasts, which keep the capsule healthy and maintain a supportive yet flexible structure. In a frozen shoulder, this typical collagen structure is disrupted by the gradual fibrosis of this connective tissue membrane and thickening of the adjacent synovial membrane. These fibrotic changes are accompanied by inflammation, angiogenesis/neovascularization, and neo-innervation. As a result, joint volume is reduced, and the capsule's stiffness increases, leading to restricted movements and pain.

Thus, a frozen shoulder is characterized by tissue fibrosis of the shoulder capsule, likely triggered by an immune response and modulated by cytokines, growth factors, and enzymes. Of these enzymes, matrix metalloproteinases (MMPs) play a particularly important role. MMPs are involved in the breakdown of the extracellular matrix. *Tissue inhibitors of metalloproteinases* (TIMPs) inhibit the activity of MMPs. A good balance between the two is crucial, as MMPs (and their inhibitors, the TIMPs) regulate matrix remodeling, which becomes dysregulated in frozen shoulder [213].

Frozen shoulder affects about 2–5% of the population [214, 215], typically between the ages of 40 and 65, with women being slightly more affected than men.

F. Struyf, *Shoulder Pain*, https://doi.org/10.1007/978-3-031-82228-5_14

There is a characteristic peak around the age of 50 [216]. Frozen shoulder is, therefore, a common shoulder condition associated with pain and progressive loss of shoulder mobility.

In theory, a frozen shoulder can be classified as either primary or secondary. Primary refers to an unknown cause, while secondary is linked to trauma, surgery, or other pathologies such as RCRSP. The underlying cause of the entire process can sometimes be a minor injury or accident, a shoulder surgery, or, in some cases, no specific cause can be identified.

Frozen shoulder has been associated with a range of comorbidities, including cardiovascular diseases, Parkinson's disease, stroke, hyperthyroidism, and especially diabetes mellitus, where the incidence of frozen shoulder can reach up to nearly 60% [88, 213]. Additionally, in individuals with diabetes, frozen shoulder tends to last longer and have a worse prognosis than in those without diabetes. This association is likely multifactorial due to the presence of chronic low-grade inflammation in people with diabetes and the presence of *advanced glycation end products* (binding of glucose to proteins, AGEs). AGEs contribute to fibrosis and inflammation in various organ systems of people with diabetes. First, AGEs form cross-links between collagen molecules, leading to resistance to proteolysis and reduced tissue compliance. Second, AGEs stimulate the production of pro-inflammatory and pro-fibrotic cytokines and immune cells. Lastly, AGEs can also contribute to the imbalanced MMP and/or TIMP activity observed in all diabetic organ systems.

Other risk factors associated with frozen shoulder include hyperlipidemia, Dupuytren's disease, autoimmune diseases, smoking, obesity, and a low level of physical activity. These conditions are all linked to chronic low-grade inflammation, which has also been associated with frozen shoulder [217]. Several theories connect frozen shoulder to these conditions. Additionally, it is quite mysterious that once you have had a frozen shoulder, you are unlikely to get it again in the same shoulder. So, the good news is that you can only develop a frozen shoulder a maximum of two times in your life.

The term "frozen shoulder" primarily refers to the stiffness that develops in the joint as the condition progresses. A frozen shoulder typically begins with a painful onset, followed by severe loss of movement and stiffness, which gives the condition its name. Often, but not always, a frozen shoulder goes through several typical phases: the *freezing* phase, the *frozen* phase, and the *thawing* phase. That final phase sounds like good news to many patients.

During the *freezing* phase, the patient mainly experiences a lot of pain, both at rest and during shoulder movements. As a result of this pain, the range of motion of the shoulder will quickly decrease. This is likely due to an increased activity of myofibroblasts, cells that lie between fibroblasts and smooth muscle cells. Fibroblasts are responsible for the production of connective tissue, but in the case of myofibroblasts, they may also have a function like that of muscles, allowing them to contract, which could explain the rapid restriction in the first weeks after the onset of a frozen shoulder. The *freezing* phase can vary from a few weeks to an average of 9 months. This phase is characterized by an inflammatory synovial reaction and hypervascular synovitis.

During the *frozen* phase, the pain usually subsides, and stiffness becomes more prominent. Subsequently, the connective tissue structure surrounding the shoulder—the joint capsule—will become much stiffer, and the range of motion will further decrease. Intra-articularly, there is ongoing synovitis and progressive capsular contracture. During arthroscopy, hypervascular synovitis and a loss of axillary fold can be observed. This phase can again last 4 to 9 months.

Finally, the last phase occurs, the thawing phase, in which there is a gradual improvement in stiffness. Biopsy of patients with stage 3 frozen shoulder shows dense, hypercellular collagen tissue with a thin synovial layer, like other fibrosing conditions. This phase can again last several months.

In summary, a frozen shoulder usually progresses through three overlapping stages: the inflammatory or *freezing* phase (stage 1 with mostly pain and initial loss of motion), the *frozen* phase (stage 2 with mainly stiffness), and, finally, the *thawing* phase (stage 3, where symptoms gradually improve). However, not all patients progress neatly through the different stages. In particular, the last phase can last longer than hoped. One assumes that a frozen shoulder will fully recover on its own, supposedly being self-limiting, even if no treatment is done. Unfortunately, while it is typically stated that a frozen shoulder is a self-limiting condition (recovery after approximately 1.5 years), various studies have shown that stiffness and pain persist much longer [216, 218] and that there is no evidence of full recovery without guided treatment [219].

How Do You Recognize a Frozen Shoulder?

A frozen shoulder is primarily characterized by pain, especially at night and during sudden or unexpected movements, along with a general loss of shoulder mobility [142]. The patient with a frozen shoulder experiences diffuse shoulder pain, meaning the pain spreads across the entire shoulder and radiates to the chest, upper arm, and sometimes even to the elbow. Pain intensity is often higher in patients with the most severe restrictions. Pain is mainly localized to the anterior shoulder (dermatomes C5–C6) and rarely extended beyond the distal third of the arm [220]. However, other shoulder conditions can present a similar picture, so this alone is not specific enough.

In the absence of movement restriction, it would be difficult to distinguish it from a patient with rotator cuff-related shoulder pain. However, in a frozen shoulder, the pain is often described as constant, deep, and usually quite severe. It only becomes clear that it is a frozen shoulder when the shoulder stiffens. One of the typical restrictions in the shoulder is external rotation range of motion, likely due to the involvement of the coracohumeral ligament.

In the international literature [143], a frozen shoulder is defined as a loss of shoulder mobility (specifically in the glenohumeral joint) greater than 25% in at least two movement planes and more than 50% in terms of external rotation with the arm at the side, compared to the unaffected side. The movement restriction must be stable or worsening for at least 1 month (Table 14.1).

Table 14.1 Clinical presentation of a frozen shoulder

Including characteristics	Excluding characteristics
Average age between 40 and 65 years	
Slow progressive pattern of increasing pain and stiffness	
Pain and stiffness interfere with sleep, ADL, and reaching in stage 1	External rotation is limited with a hard end feel (e.g., osteoarthritis or posterior luxation)
Glenohumeral mobility is limited in all directions	Passive range of motion is normal
Glenohumeral external rotation is the most restricted	Painful abduction without a decrease in external rotation ROM
Glenohumeral rotations decrease in ROM with increasing abduction	Glenohumeral rotation ROM increases with increasing abduction
Passive movements towards their end range produce typical pain	Positive upper-limb nerve test

Assessing shoulder movement in patients with severe pain can be challenging. What seems like a loss of mobility may actually be due to the patient's self-limiting behaviors caused by pain or fear. To get a clearer picture, it is helpful to evaluate movement in different positions with varying levels of support. For instance, the key movement of external rotation might appear reduced when the patient is standing. However, it should also be assessed while the patient is lying down, with support for the arm and trunk. A significant difference in range of motion (ROM) in these positions is more likely to indicate fear of movement rather than actual capsular restriction. Assessment of the cervical spine is also essential to rule out potential cervicogenic pathology, such as nerve root irritation causing radicular pain. This will be discussed in detail in the relevant chapter.

One aspect that has not received much attention is the role of chronic or persistent pain. Individuals with characteristics of anxiety and depression are at higher risk for prolonged symptoms and a poorer prognosis [221, 222]. This suggests that frozen shoulder is likely not an isolated musculoskeletal condition but rather the result of a complex interaction of multiple processes.

In addition to the previously mentioned interactions, a frozen shoulder is also a long-term condition that often falls under the category of chronic pain. Various mechanisms in the brain adapt due to ongoing pain, as is known in chronic pain conditions. Therefore, it is thought that these changes—referred to as central sensitization—may contribute to prolonged shoulder pain and potentially play a larger role in frozen shoulder than previously considered [223–225]. Although central sensitization in frozen shoulder has not been extensively studied and remains speculative, it could explain why some patients are resistant to current interventions and might benefit from a different approach.

15 Glenohumeral Instability

Throughout evolution, the shoulder has become the most mobile joint in the human body. However, the incredible mobility of the shoulder joint also has a downside: reduced stability.

Our glenohumeral capsule, bony congruence, ligaments, labrum, and surrounding muscles all work to provide shoulder stability. The shoulder joint must constantly balance mobility and stability, but sometimes this balance can fail, for example, when one of the aforementioned structures is injured. This can lead to glenohumeral instability, which is often defined as an abnormal increase in glenohumeral translation that can cause symptoms ranging from pain, subluxation, to complete dislocation of the humeral head.

Instability should not be confused with laxity. Laxity refers to excessive movement in the joint without any associated symptoms. Individuals with laxity may be able to manage it and may not experience any discomfort.

Approximately 72% of all shoulder dislocations are reported in men, particularly in younger men under the age of 20 [226]. The incidence rates indeed show a peak in younger individuals and another peak in those over 70 years old. In this latter group, the cause is likely a reduction in rotator cuff function, combined with an increased incidence of falls.

The majority of dislocation mechanisms are indeed related to a fall on the shoulder (ca. 60%), roughly split 50/50 between accidents at home and those occurring during a sport or hobby [227].

What Is Glenohumeral Instability?

In this chapter, we discuss the unstable shoulder, which can progress to subluxation or even luxation in extreme cases. In the introduction, you already read about the static and dynamic stabilizers. Each of them plays a role in the stability of our shoulder and can be a factor in instability. Instability can occur in the anterior, posterior, or in more than two directions (i.e., multidirectional instability).

F. Struyf, *Shoulder Pain*, https://doi.org/10.1007/978-3-031-82228-5_15

The mechanism leading to glenohumeral instability is often a dislocation (in about 83% of instability patients) [228]. For posterior instability, this figure is much lower, and in most cases, the patient does not even recall an incident [229].

To ensure that researchers and clinicians are looking at the same type of injury, a classification system seems necessary. Shoulder instability is now commonly divided into different types, originating from the Stanmore Triangle Classification System. The Stanmore Triangle uses three classifications of shoulder instability.

Glenohumeral Shoulder Instability Type 1

Patients classified as type 1 have experienced trauma and, as a result, exhibit structural injuries. There are various types of traumas that can lead to shoulder instability. First, we refer to dislocations of the joint. These patients do not display abnormal muscle patterns. The most common direction for a shoulder dislocation is anterior, for example, due to a direct fall on the shoulder or following a torsion. Anterior dislocations account for about 90% of all shoulder dislocations [230]. Posterior dislocations, for instance, from a fall on a horizontally adducted arm, occur in only a small percentage (up to 4%) of all dislocations.

Another reported mechanism for a posterior dislocation is epileptic seizures. The most common structural bone injuries include a Hill-Sachs lesion or a (bony) Bankart lesion. A Hill-Sachs lesion is caused by the impact of the glenoid on the humeral head, resulting in a "dent" in the humeral head. A bony Bankart lesion, on the other hand, is characterized by a fracture of the anteroinferior glenoid. The labrum will also be affected. Typical soft tissue injuries that can occur with anterior dislocations include labral Bankart lesions, where the labrum detaches from the anteroinferior glenoid. Additionally, tears of the inferior glenohumeral ligament (*humeral avulsion glenohumeral ligament*, HAGL) or variations of different labral injuries may occur.

Glenohumeral Shoulder Instability Type 2

Patients classified as type 2 have not experienced trauma but still have (less extensive than type 1) a structural injury. They also do not exhibit abnormal muscle patterns. These shoulders can dislocate or subluxate during normal everyday activities. In this group, the shoulder's active and/or passive stabilizers are subjected to repeated microtrauma. Over time, this causes tissue damage and pain. Some shoulders have a congenital anatomy that predisposes them to a shoulder dislocation (e.g., twisted humeral head or labral abnormalities), while other patients do not have congenital abnormalities, such as many overhead athletes.

The structural injuries can again be bony or more soft tissue in nature, as described above. Type 2 shoulder instability also includes hypermobile patients or those with connective tissue disorders.

Joint laxity can be associated with generalized hypermobility, but this is not always the case. To identify generalized joint laxity, the Beighton score is useful [231, 232]. Using this scoring system, we assign each individual a score between 0 and 9 by checking the following characteristics of hypermobility:

- Left and right pinky finger hyperextension more than 90 degrees (1 point per side)
- Bringing the thumb to the ventral side of the forearm during wrist flexion (1 point per side)
- More than 10 degrees of hyperextension in the elbow (1 point per side)
- Bending forward with straight legs and placing both flat hands on the ground (1 point)
- Hyperextension at the knees, observed while standing (1 point per side)

According to the Beighton method, a score of 5 or higher indicates generalized hypermobility.

A relationship was found between generalized joint hypermobility and a history of glenohumeral joint instability, with participants who had instability showing higher total Beighton Scale scores and those scoring 2 or above being over twice as likely to have experienced previous instability episodes compared to those with lower scores [233].

Glenohumeral Shoulder Instability Type 3

Type 3 shoulder instability involves patients who have not experienced trauma or structural injury but do experience symptoms due to abnormal muscle contractions (weakened or with reduced control). This is a more complex problem that occurs less frequently than type 1 or type 2. The cause of this instability type is still poorly researched and can vary greatly.

However, we prefer not to use the term “abnormal contraction” as it seems too vague and untreatable, but for now, we must rely on it. By “abnormal contraction,” we mean an unfavorable pattern of muscle contractions that do not center the humeral head but instead pull it out of its socket. It is suspected that primarily the large and strong muscles, such as the pectoralis major muscle and latissimus dorsi muscle, are responsible for this. The pectoralis major muscle pulls the humerus anteriorly out of the socket, while the latissimus dorsi muscle tends to pull the humeral head posteriorly out of the socket.

Strong muscle contractions can pull the shoulder out of the socket, as we have seen in patients with epileptic seizures. However, most abnormal muscle contractions result in a subtle sense of instability or subluxation, which can eventually lead to pain.

Of course, our patients do not always fit neatly into one category, and you will frequently encounter combinations. For example, think of a patient who has experienced trauma (type 1) but already exhibits structural injuries as a result of nontraumatic instability (type 2).

How Do You Recognize Glenohumeral Instability?

Generally, glenohumeral instability is associated with a feeling of instability or looseness in the shoulder, sometimes describing the shoulder as "wobbly." Patients may also report pain or experience neurovascular consequences. Additionally, kinesiophobia may be present. Kinesiophobia is an intense fear of movement or physical activity. During the patient history, the patient may describe experiencing subluxations, apprehension (avoidance behavior), or a sensation of shoulder instability. These symptoms typically occur at the end of their range of motion.

In cases of anterior instability, pain may also occur, for example, in the anterior region near the long head of the biceps brachii muscle. Fatigue in the entire arm is also a commonly recurring symptom, and in posterior instability, pain is often one of the typical symptoms.

Questions we always want to have answered include those about the mechanism of injury, the patient's age, the direction of the instability, the provoking movements, the impact on their life, and the possible presence of hypermobility.

Glenohumeral Instability Type 1/Anterior Shoulder Dislocation

In addition to what an X-ray can reveal, there are also clinical signs that may indicate a shoulder dislocation. A dislocation primarily causes significant pain. The patient will also avoid moving the shoulder and may not allow passive examination. Furthermore, the shoulder may show altered contours. The normal rounded profile of the deltoid muscle may appear angular, with a visible subacromial notch (sulcus).

Glenohumeral Instability Type 2

During history taking, patients with type 2 shoulder instability will report shoulder dislocation or subluxation or a feeling of instability without a history of trauma. Moreover, these patients are often able to relocate their shoulder on their own (or with minimal assistance). These are the clear type 2 instabilities. However, there are also many patients with more subtle symptoms, such as clicking, a slight feeling of instability, laxity, or some pain. These latter symptoms can resemble a rotator cuff-related problem and often co-occur. For instance, type 2 shoulder instability can be the underlying cause of chronic rotator cuff tendinopathy.

Anterior instability is typically characterized by a positive *apprehension* (sensitivity 65.6% and specificity 95.4%), *relocation* (sensitivity 65% and specificity 90%), and *release test* (sensitivity 82% and specificity 86%), where the patient reports typical symptoms such as a feeling of instability, fear of movement, or clicking when the arm is placed in an abduction and external rotation position [146]. It is crucial to interpret these tests based on fear or avoidance behavior rather than pain [234].

The load and shift test [235] and the sulcus sign [236] are used to assess the degree of laxity in a joint, not to diagnose instability. Additionally, the reliability of assessing movement and measuring laxity is limited due to the risk of false negatives, as patients may be unable to fully relax during the tests. Therefore, these tests should be used with caution. Since people with generalized laxity are at a higher risk of multidirectional instability, the above tests are frequently used in diagnosing multidirectional instability. Examination of patients with multidirectional instability often reveals generalized muscle atrophy and scapular dyskinesis.

In the case of posterior instability, clinicians must rely on a combination of a thorough patient history, including the injury mechanism, symptoms, and recognition of risk factors [237, 238]. With a positive *likelihood* ratio of 19, the posterior apprehension test can be of additional value. Be aware, where the apprehension sign was so important in anterior instability, pain will now be a key determining factor in posterior instability. The use of a single orthopedic special test is not recommended for posterior instability.

Glenohumeral Instability Type 3

Patients with glenohumeral instability type 3 are on average often young women in their 20s with hypermobility (often initially classified as type 2). This group exhibits not only anterior instability but also posterior or inferior instability, leading to multidirectional instability. Additionally, psychosocial factors may play a larger role in these patients than in other instability patients. Some suspect that these factors underlie abnormal muscle patterns, though this has not yet been scientifically proven. It is possible that type 3 shoulder instability makes the patient feel unhappy, anxious, or worried. This presents an area for further research.

The clinical examination of type 3 shoulder instability is partly based on visual observation during the active movement assessment. For example, patients may exhibit jerky movements, as if a car were driving on square wheels. Others may attempt to perform the entire movement with excessive force, while still others display an abnormal scapulothoracic rhythm, where the scapula rotates upward or is lifted prematurely.

The Apprehension, Relocation, and Release Test

For the *apprehension, relocation, and release test*, the patient lies supine on the treatment table with the affected arm hanging off the edge of the table. The arm is brought into 90 degrees of abduction, with the elbow in 90 degrees of flexion. Make sure that the humerus rests over treatment table, but the humeral head remains on the table. As the practitioner, stand on the affected side, facing the patient, and grasp the patient's elbow with your contralateral hand. Move the shoulder into maximum external rotation and horizontal abduction. Ensure that you do not support the upper arm but allow it to move backward freely.

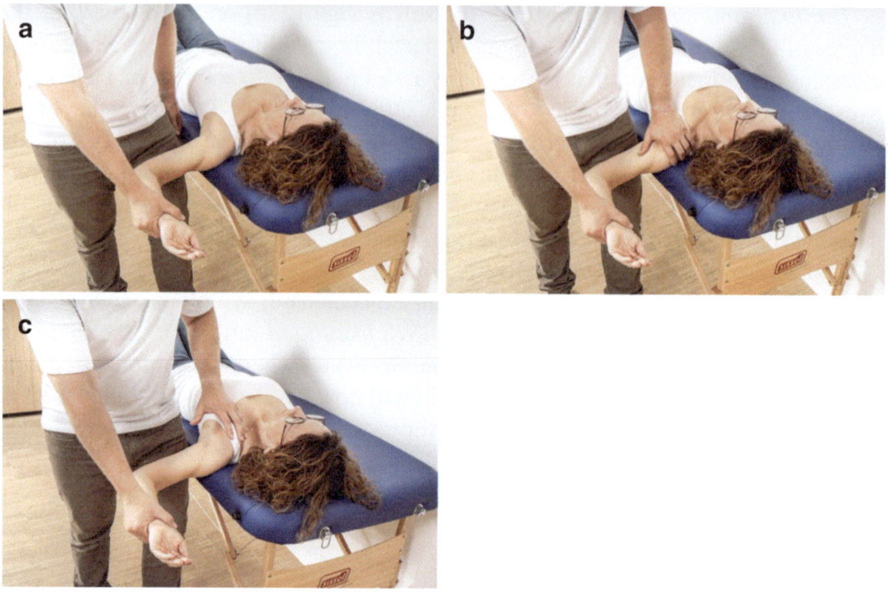

Fig. 15.1 (**a–c**) The apprehension, relocation, and release test

The test is positive if the patient expresses recognizable fear of subluxation or if there is a click or activation of the pectoralis major muscle. This is the *apprehension test*. Then maintain the position from the apprehension test and apply an anterior-to-posterior translation on the humeral head with your ipsilateral hand. The test is positive if the previously mentioned symptoms disappear or lessen. This is the *relocation test.*

Finally, remove your ipsilateral hand from the humeral head. The test is positive if the symptoms return. This is *the release test*, also known as the *surprise test* (Fig. 15.1a–c).

The Load and Shift Test

For the *load and shift test*, the patient sits on the treatment table with their hands resting on their thighs. Using your ipsilateral hand, grasp the humerus as proximally as possible, while your contralateral hand stabilizes the scapula. You can then ask the patient to perform an isometric contraction into abduction (e.g., against your leg while asking to clench a fist) to center the humeral head (*load*).

Next, ask the patient to relax the shoulder, and with the ipsilateral hand, you can then push/pull the humeral head forward or backward (*shift*). The test is considered positive when there is increased movement according to the following classification: Grade 0, minimal translation; Grade 1, translation within the glenoid socket;

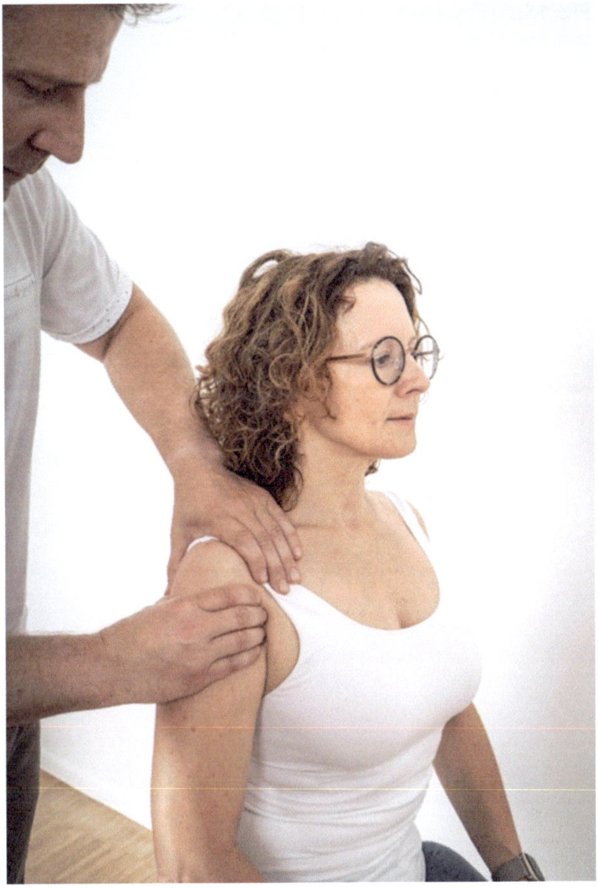

Fig. 15.2 The load and shift test

Grade 2, translation to the edge of the glenoid with spontaneous reduction; and Grade 3, translation beyond the edge with persistent dislocation (Fig. 15.2).

The Sulcus Sign

For the sulcus sign test, have the patient sit on the treatment table and the affected arm hanging relaxed. Stabilize the shoulder with your contralateral hand by placing your palm on the acromion and palpating the joint space with your thumb and index finger. With your ipsilateral hand, grasp the patient's affected arm just proximal to the humeral epicondyles and apply a downward traction on the humerus.

The test is positive if a sulcus appears between the humeral head and the inferior border of the acromion. This can be further classified as grade 0, no sulcus; grade 1, a sulcus one finger-width wide; and grade 2, a sulcus two fingers-width wide. This test can also be performed with the patient standing, leaning forward on the treatment table with the arm hanging beside the body (Fig. 15.3).

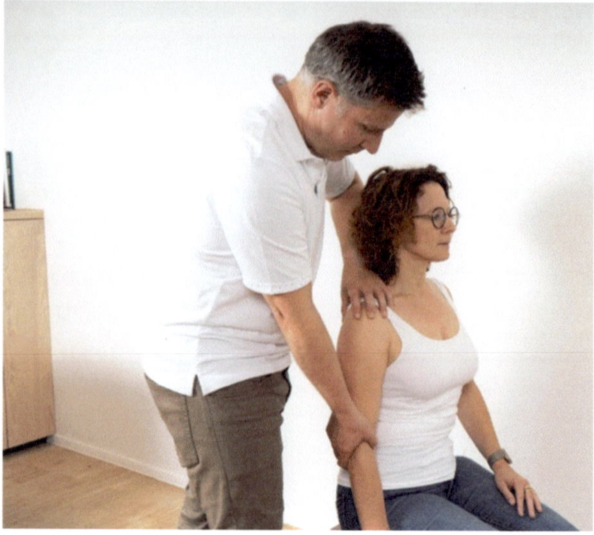

Fig. 15.3 The sulcus sign test

Acromioclavicular, Sternoclavicular, and Clavicular Conditions

16

The acromioclavicular joint (AC joint), which connects the upper extremity to the axial skeleton, can be involved in shoulder issues, particularly in individuals in their 20s and 30s and in athletes. The SC joint, which connects the shoulder blade to the rest of the body, has an interarticular disc that increases stability and acts as a cushion between the bone ends.

The AC joint connects the upper extremity to the axial skeleton. It is estimated that about 9% of all shoulder problems involve the AC joint and around 11% when the patient is seen in the emergency department [239]. The majority of these injuries occur in individuals in their 20s and 30s [240], typically athletes, with men being two to five times more likely to suffer from an AC injury than women [241]. Most injuries occur during contact sports such as rugby, wrestling, and hockey [241].

The sternoclavicular (SC) joint is the only joint that connects the shoulder blade to the rest of the body via the clavicle. The stability of the joint is further enhanced by an interarticular disc that divides the joint cavity into two parts. This fibrocartilaginous disc not only improves stability but also acts as a cushion between the bone ends.

What Is an Acromioclavicular Disorder?

Acromioclavicular (AC) disorders can arise from traumatic events, such as a direct fall onto the shoulder [240], or from degenerative conditions such as osteoarthritis, osteolysis of the distal clavicle, or post-traumatic arthritis [242]. However, direct trauma is the most common injury mechanism: a fall or a blow to the shoulder with the arm in an adducted position.

An indirect force on the AC joint can also cause injury, for example, from a fall onto the elbow or an outstretched arm, which can drive the humerus proximally against the acromion [240].

F. Struyf, *Shoulder Pain*, https://doi.org/10.1007/978-3-031-82228-5_16

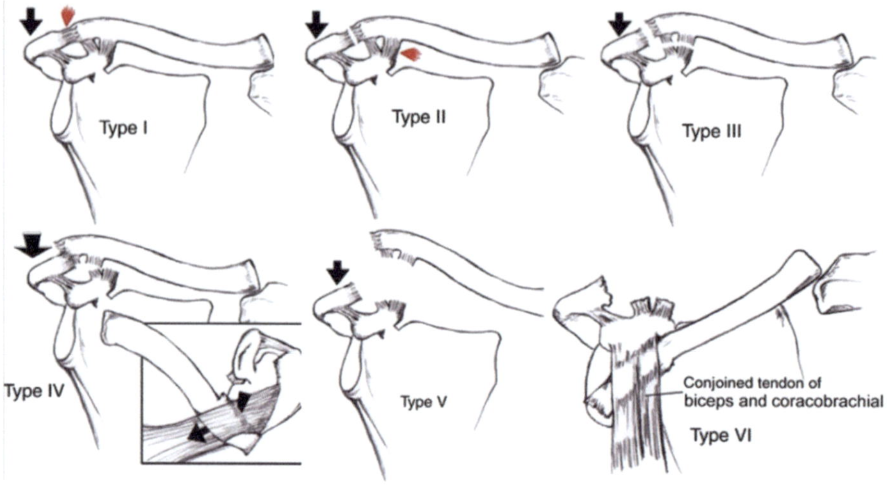

Fig. 16.1 Rockwood classification of acromioclavicular injuries, Types I–VI. (Figure reproduced with permission from Lasanianos NG, Kanakaris NK, Giannoudis PV, eds. Trauma and Orthopaedic Classifications. London, UK: Springer-Verlag London; 2015:3–6)

One of the most commonly used and accepted classifications for various AC injuries is the Rockwood classification (Fig. 16.1). The Rockwood classification describes six types of AC injuries [243].

Type I involves a mild sprain of the AC ligament. In Type II, the AC ligament is torn, and the first strain occurs on the coracoclavicular ligament. Radiographically, not much will be visible in Type I, while in Type II, a slight elevation of the clavicle relative to the acromion can be seen. In Type III, the AC joint is dislocated, and the coracoclavicular ligaments and joint capsule are also torn. Here, the clavicle shifts upward, while in Type IV, the clavicle dislocates posteriorly, with involvement of the trapezius muscle. In Type V, the clavicle dislocates further upward, and the scapula drops downward due to the detachment of both the trapezius and deltoid muscles. Finally, in Type VI, the clavicle moves downward. These types can also be combined with a fracture of the clavicle or injuries to the sternoclavicular joint.

The acromioclavicular joint can also present with instability, but it is reported in only 3–4 people per 100,000 in the general population each year [244]. The cause is usually traumatic. Atraumatic AC instability is very rare.

How Do You Recognize an Acromioclavicular Disorder?

A thorough medical history is crucial for identifying an AC injury. If the patient mentions an accident or fall, a trauma analysis should clarify whether the patient landed on the shoulder. Patients with an AC injury usually complain of pain at the top of the shoulder around the AC joint. Unlike most shoulder conditions, the pain is directly localized over the joint or in the surrounding muscular area (trapezius muscle, deltoid muscle) [242, 245]. Additionally, swelling or deformity around the AC joint may be observed [246]. The pain often occurs during functional activities that compress or stretch the AC joint, such as washing the opposite armpit or fastening a bra [242].

Various diagnostic tests have been described for diagnosing AC joint disorders, but their diagnostic value is generally weak [246]. Many of these tests need to be used in combination to increase the *likelihood* ratio: the Paxinos test combined with the O'Brien test provides a specificity and sensitivity of over 90% [247]. Palpation for local AC tenderness has a high sensitivity (96%) but low specificity (10%) [234, 248].

The Paxinos Test

For the Paxinos test (Fig. 16.2), the patient sits upright in a chair with the arm at their side. The therapist stands behind the patient, placing their hand over the

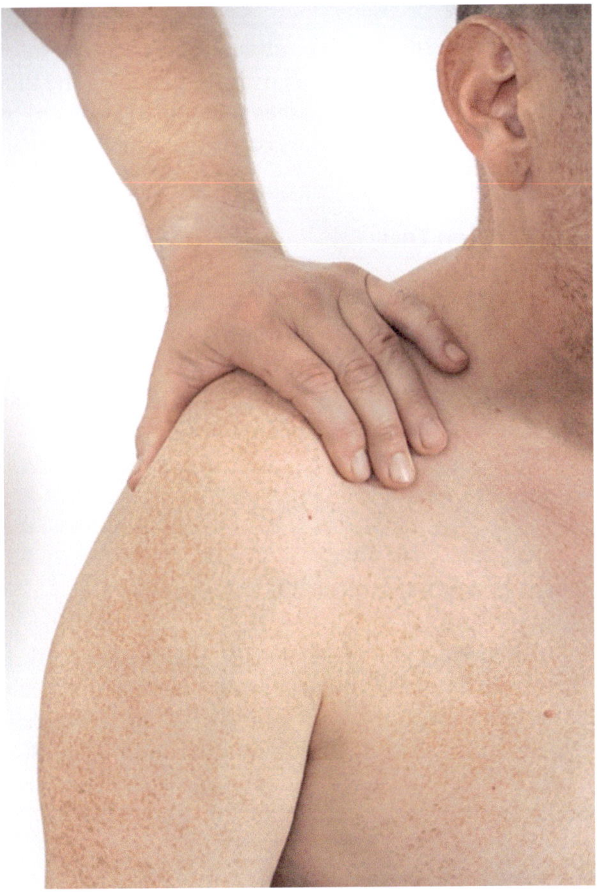

Fig. 16.2 The Paxinos test

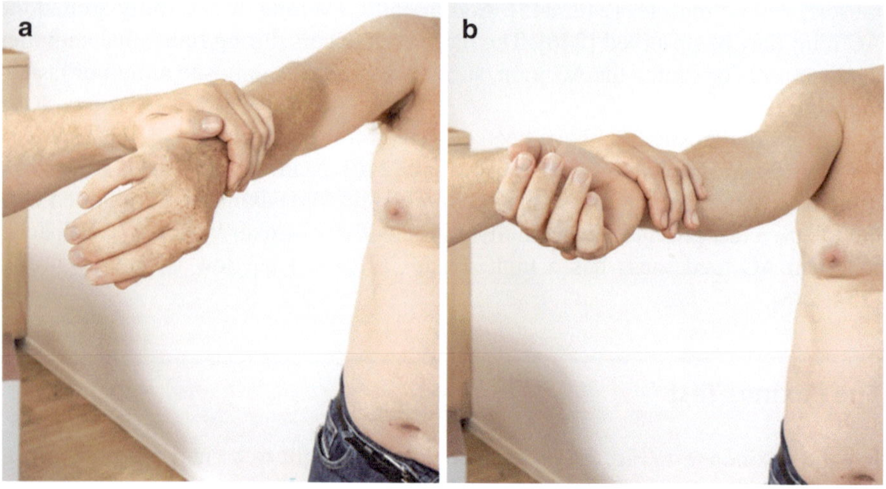

Fig. 16.3 (**a, b**) The O'Brien test

shoulder, with the thumb positioned at the postero-inferior side of the acromion and the index and middle fingers over the clavicle. The thumb and fingers apply opposing pressure: the thumb pushes forward and upward, while the fingers push downward and backward. The test is positive if it causes pain at the AC joint.

The O'Brien Test

For the O'Brien test (Fig. 16.3a, b), the patient sits upright in a chair or stands, with the arm in 90 degrees of forward flexion, 10 degrees of horizontal adduction, and full internal rotation. As the examiner, you apply downward pressure on the patient's forearm while they try to maintain their arm in the same position. The test is then repeated with the arm in a neutral position.

The test is positive if it causes pain at the AC joint in the first position, with less discomfort in the second position.

What Is a Sternoclavicular Disorder?

Injuries to the sternoclavicular (SC) joint are relatively rare, accounting for about 3% of all shoulder girdle injuries. Anterior dislocations are more common than posterior dislocations, with a ratio of 20 to 1. Typically, clavicle fractures or acromioclavicular joint dislocations occur before the SC joint is affected. The usual cause is direct lateral compression of the shoulder, such as from a fall onto the side of the shoulder.

This type of injury is commonly seen in sports like martial arts, horseback riding, cycling, and rugby. When the SC joint dislocates, it moves in the opposite direction of the applied force. For example, a fall on the back will push the acromion anteriorly and move the clavicle posteriorly in the SC joint. This can sometimes be particularly dangerous due to the vital structures located behind the SC joint. Several important structures are near the joint, including the esophagus, trachea, lungs, pleura, brachial plexus, and major arteries and veins. Posterior dislocation can, therefore, be potentially life-threatening if severe.

Fortunately, this is quite rare, with anterior dislocations being much more common. These can occur without trauma and often cause only mild discomfort. Atraumatic SC instability is again very rare and strongly associated with hypermobility syndromes [249].

How Do You Recognize a Sternoclavicular Disorder?

In the initial examination of a posterior SC joint dislocation, the focus should be on ruling out life-threatening injury. Symptoms such as an abnormal sound caused by impaired airflow in the airways during breathing, bluish discoloration, speech difficulties, pulsating blood vessels, and neurological symptoms may necessitate immediate hospitalization.

If these symptoms are absent, the joint can be further examined. The pain is usually of a localized nature and may gradually worsen over time. Anterior SC dislocation causes visible deformity, while posterior dislocation removes the usual prominence over the inside of the collarbone. Local swelling, crepitus, and pain with movement, especially horizontal flexion, may also be present.

There is insufficient research to support the use of specific tests in the assessment of the SC joint. The protraction test combined with local palpation is described as a reliable method for diagnosing degenerative SC pathology [250]. However, it remains unclear whether this combination is also effective in patients with SC instability.

Finally, musculoskeletal tumors of the distal clavicle and proximal acromion are uncommon but should be considered when accompanied by night pain, pain at rest, or systemic symptoms.

What Is a Clavicular Disorder?

When we think of a clavicular disorder, clavicle fractures come to mind first. The most common mechanism is a fall onto an outstretched arm or directly onto the shoulder. In cases of suspected clavicle fracture, a neurovascular and pulmonary examination should always be conducted due to the proximity of important structures such as the subclavian artery, parts of the brachial plexus, and the upper lobe of the lung.

How Do You Recognize a Clavicular Disorder?

Typically, there is a cracking sensation at the time of injury, accompanied by immediate pain at the fracture site and rapid swelling. Visible deformity may also occur. Fractures of the proximal and middle third of the clavicle account for approximately 80% of these injuries. Notably, fractures at the very proximal end of the clavicle can be misdiagnosed as sternoclavicular dislocations. In younger individuals, particularly those up to 25 years old, it is essential to consider the possibility of epiphyseal injury in this area. Imaging options, such as X-rays and CT scans, can be critical in accurately diagnosing the type and extent of the fracture, ensuring appropriate treatment and preventing complications.

Glenohumeral Osteoarthritis 17

The population is aging, and this has a significant impact on the incidence of glenohumeral osteoarthritis. According to the most recent UN population projections (World Population Prospects: the 2024 Revision; https://population.un.org/wpp/), the number of people aged 60 or older is expected to rise from 1.2 million to 2.1 billion by 2050, doubling and even tripling for those aged 80 and above. In addition, osteoarthritis ranks among the top 5 (for women) and top 10 (for men) most disabling diseases in people aged 60 and over. Furthermore, the rates of obesity and diabetes are also increasing. Altogether, it is often suggested that the incidence of osteoarthritis will rise dramatically in the coming decades.

It is estimated that 2–5% of all shoulder patients have glenohumeral osteoarthritis [251]. Moreover, degenerative changes in the glenohumeral joint are increasingly found in patients with shoulder pain, reaching up to 17%. But these changes are not always the cause of the complaint [252, 253]. They are also often related to the presence of massive rotator cuff tears. The prevalence of glenohumeral osteoarthritis clearly increases with age, from 1.8% in individuals in their 40s to 27.5% in those in their 80s [254, 255]. Glenohumeral osteoarthritis is thus a common cause of shoulder pain in adults over 65 years old.

What Is Glenohumeral Osteoarthritis?

Glenohumeral osteoarthritis is characterized by degeneration of the joint cartilage and subchondral bone, as well as damage to the ligaments, muscles, and synovium around the joint. As a result, a narrowing of the glenohumeral joint occurs. The pathogenesis of glenohumeral osteoarthritis is quite complex and not yet fully understood. It appears that several factors contribute to joint damage. In the glenohumeral joint, focal or general cartilage loss and subsequent subchondral bone sclerosis are most pronounced in the upper two-thirds of the humeral head [256].

The most common bone change in glenohumeral osteoarthritis is likely the formation of osteophytes. Osteophytes mainly develop in areas where there is capsular

F. Struyf, *Shoulder Pain*, https://doi.org/10.1007/978-3-031-82228-5_17

traction, particularly on the anterior and inferior sides of the humeral head and inferiorly around the glenoid [257]. Osteophytes lead to joint stiffness and are sometimes seen as the joint's natural way of preventing pain by forming arthrodesis.

On the other hand, there are theories that attribute pain specifically to these osteophytes. However, it is important to remember that distinguishing between causes and effects based on radiological imaging can be challenging. Not all patients exhibit the same morphological characteristics. In the past, osteoarthritis was described as cartilage disease primarily caused by joint wear, often due to aging. Today, we know it is a condition that affects the entire joint, including the surrounding tissues. The pathogenesis of glenohumeral osteoarthritis is now seen as part of a larger process, involving specific, nonspecific, systemic, or local factors. The progression of glenohumeral osteoarthritis is likely influenced by a combination of genetic, behavioral, and environmental factors.

Nonspecific General Risk Factors for Glenohumeral Osteoarthritis

Aging is likely the most significant etiological risk factor for developing glenohumeral osteoarthritis. As we age, the density of our cartilage decreases, making it more vulnerable [258]. However, hereditary factors also play a role. Some researchers estimate that as many as 65% of patients with osteoarthritis have a genetic predisposition [259].

While weight is typically considered a risk factor for weight-bearing joints such as the hips and knees, its role in shoulder osteoarthritis is less clear but still significant. Increased adipose tissue can contribute to systemic inflammation through the secretion of pro-inflammatory cytokines, which may negatively affect cartilage health in all joints, including the shoulder. This inflammatory environment can accelerate cartilage degradation and promote the onset of osteoarthritis. Furthermore, excess body fat may alter joint biomechanics, potentially leading to increased stress on the shoulder joint and exacerbating wear and tear. Addressing body fat levels may therefore play a crucial role in managing shoulder osteoarthritis and preserving cartilage integrity [260, 261].

Nonspecific Local Risk Factors for Glenohumeral Osteoarthritis

Where it was once believed that excessive joint loading could lead to increased wear, it is now more widely accepted that an appropriate amount of movement and load can actually prevent cartilage degeneration [262]. The word "appropriate" is key here. On the one hand, insufficient load weakens our muscles and joints, while on the other hand, excessive load can accelerate the progression of osteoarthritis.

Excessive shoulder loading often involves heavy, overhead movements. Consequently, weightlifters and certain throwing athletes are at a slightly higher risk of developing glenohumeral osteoarthritis [263].

Specific Local Risk Factors for Glenohumeral Osteoarthritis

There are several shoulder conditions that increase the likelihood of developing glenohumeral osteoarthritis. First, we have shoulder instability, particularly after dislocations, both with and without surgical stabilization, where a higher degree of osteoarthritis-related damage is visible on radiological imaging. However, it is unclear whether these changes are due to direct impact injuries or persistent instability. Patients with a single glenohumeral dislocation are thought to have at least ten times the risk of developing radiological glenohumeral osteoarthritis [264] This risk increases further with multiple dislocations.

Second, fractures can damage the joint cartilage. Fractures may also trigger a cascade of inflammatory processes that lead to trauma-induced osteoarthritis, known as post-traumatic glenohumeral osteoarthritis. In addition to directly damaging the cartilage, fractures of the proximal humerus and glenoid can alter biomechanics, potentially resulting in osteoarthritis, similar to what occurs with instability.

Third, the rotator cuff may be torn to the extent that the humeral head undergoes cranial migration, which can lead to degenerative changes in the glenohumeral joint. This is most noticeable as selective degeneration on the superior side of the glenoid. This condition is referred to as rotator cuff arthropathy.

Lastly, cartilage degeneration is sometimes attributed to various forms of the glenoid or acromion, brachial plexus palsy, or the Milwaukee shoulder. Milwaukee shoulder syndrome is a rare joint-destructive degenerative condition characterized by severe shoulder pain and limited motion, often linked to rotator cuff tears and advanced osteoarthritis.

Specific Systemic Risk Factors for Glenohumeral Osteoarthritis

Systemic diseases affecting the shoulder have also been reported as risk factors for glenohumeral osteoarthritis. Various forms of glenohumeral arthritis are associated with a higher risk of osteoarthritis, particularly rheumatoid arthritis, psoriatic arthritis, juvenile idiopathic arthritis, spondyloarthropathy, and lupus erythematosus. Rheumatoid arthritis is the most well-known and common of these conditions, affecting the glenohumeral joint in about half of patients with rheumatoid arthritis [265]. Furthermore, crystalline arthropathies such as gout can lead to inflammatory joint damage.

In addition to inflammatory diseases, the humeral head can be significantly impacted by avascular necrosis, commonly resulting from corticosteroid use, alcoholism, or trauma. This condition, characterized by reduced blood supply to the bone, leads to osteonecrosis and subsequently causes a loss of joint congruence. Over time, this deterioration can increase the risk of developing osteoarthritis, as the compromised structural integrity of the humeral head can accelerate cartilage wear and joint degeneration, ultimately resulting in pain and functional limitations. Only a small percentage (ca. 5%) of all patients with glenohumeral osteoarthritis are thought to have this condition [266].

Finally, endocrine diseases and neuropathic arthropathies are also described as possible causes of glenohumeral osteoarthritis. Cervical syringomyelia is responsible for 75% of neuropathic shoulder arthropathies. Other causes can include diabetes mellitus or alcoholism [267].

How Do You Recognize Glenohumeral Osteoarthritis?

During the patient history, the patient will primarily complain of a progressive, persistent pain located deep within the joint, often posteriorly. Although articular cartilage is relatively insensitive, the periarticular tissues, such as the synovium and subchondral bone, are richly innervated and therefore likely sources of nociceptive signals [268].

The patient will report tenderness along the joint line during palpation. Glenohumeral osteoarthritis causes significant pain, stiffness, reduced range of motion, functional impairment, and disability. The loss of passive motion is often most pronounced in external rotation. These patients also typically present with night pain and pain at rest. Muscle atrophy may also be evident. However, glenohumeral osteoarthritis is not the most common cause of shoulder pain. As noted, this presentation resembles that of a frozen shoulder. A patient with a frozen shoulder typically will not show any radiological abnormalities. Also, a patient suspected of having glenohumeral osteoarthritis is usually two decades older than one with a frozen shoulder. More common conditions, such as frozen shoulder, should therefore be ruled out first. As glenohumeral osteoarthritis worsens, other symptoms may develop, such as restricted movement and crepitus.

18 Neurologically Related Shoulder Conditions

Not all shoulder conditions have a musculoskeletal origin. We must always consider neurological structures in differential diagnosis, such as cervical radiculopathy, nerve injuries and compression neuropathies, hemiplegic shoulder pain after a stroke, thoracic outlet syndrome, or Parsonage-Turner syndrome.

Neuropathy refers to a condition in which there is damage, disease, or dysfunction of a nerve. Cervical radiculopathy involves nerve impairment in the neck, while hemiplegic shoulder pain is a common complication after a stroke. The Parsonage-Turner syndrome is a peripheral nervous system disorder characterized by severe pain and muscle atrophy. Recognizing these conditions is important for timely diagnosis and treatment.

What Is a Neuropathy?

A neuropathy occurs when there is damage, disease, or dysfunction of a nerve. The cause of neuropathies can be very complex, ranging from diabetic neuropathies, compression neuropathies, neuropathies caused by oncological treatments, and so on. Often, there is a clear trauma present as a cause, such as a car accident or a fall from a height resulting in neurogenic elongation. A humeral fracture that injures a nerve can also cause a neuropathy. But also, subtler traumas, such as a subluxating shoulder, can cause a peripheral neuropathy. Furthermore, a nerve injury due to shoulder surgery cannot always be ruled out.

F. Struyf, *Shoulder Pain*, https://doi.org/10.1007/978-3-031-82228-5_18

Compression neuropathies around the shoulder are not very common. Overhead athletes turn out to be a risk group, with the suprascapular nerve being the most frequently affected [269]. Examination of paresthesia, numbness, hyperalgesia, allodynia, spontaneous pain, strength deficits, and two-point discrimination are essential parts of the clinical neurological assessment. Additionally, a referral for an EMG, nerve conduction study, or imaging can provide further clarification if necessary. Unfortunately, there are no adequate neurodynamic tests available for this nerve.

Another potentially affected neurogenic structure is the brachial plexus. The causes are not always clear. In some cases, they are associated with thoracic outlet syndrome (TOS), breast cancer treatment (surgery, radiation, or chemotherapy), or a lung apex tumor (Pancoast). Differential diagnosis is crucial, as both Pancoast tumors and frozen shoulder can present with similar shoulder and arm pain, but they have vastly different underlying pathologies. One of the typical manifestations of neuropathy is increased mechanosensitivity of the nerve tissue, highlighting the importance of accurate diagnosis to guide appropriate treatment.

How Do You Recognize Neuropathy?

Neurodynamic tests have been described to assess the increased mechanosensitivity of the nervous system. In the presence of increased mechanosensitivity, neurodynamic tests are more likely to be positive. However, a negative neurodynamic test does not rule out a neurogenic injury, as increased mechanosensitivity may not be present.

Neurodynamic tests of the upper limb are commonly referred to as *upper limb tension tests* (ULTT), with specific numbering depending on the nerve being tested: the median nerve (ULNT1 and 2A; Figs. 18.1 and 18.2), radial nerve (ULNT2B; Fig. 18.3), and ulnar nerve (ULNT3; Fig. 18.4) [270]. By changing the position of the shoulder, neck, and elbow joints, we can selectively stretch a nerve.

It is important that the typical symptoms are reproduced. Differentiating from stretching of musculoskeletal structures is therefore very important.

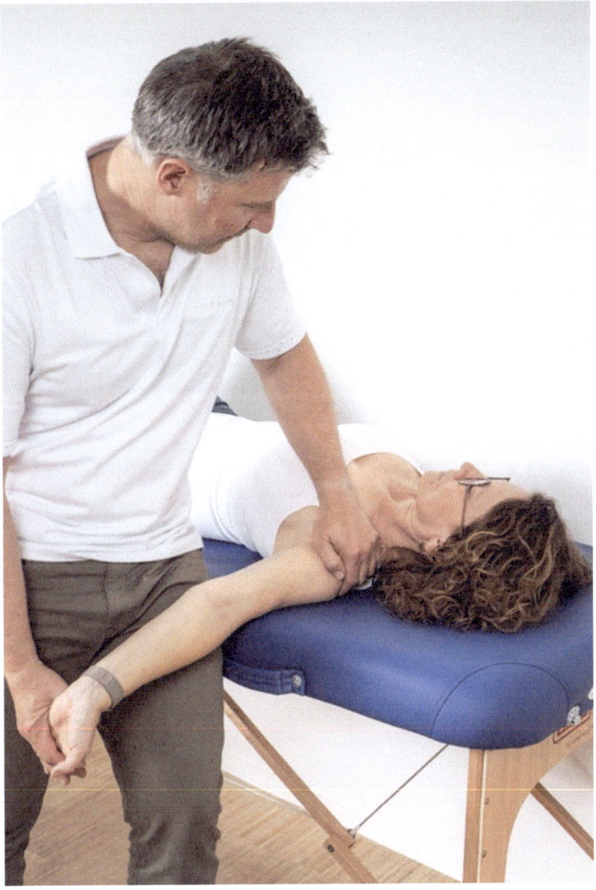

Fig. 18.1 ULNT1 median nerve

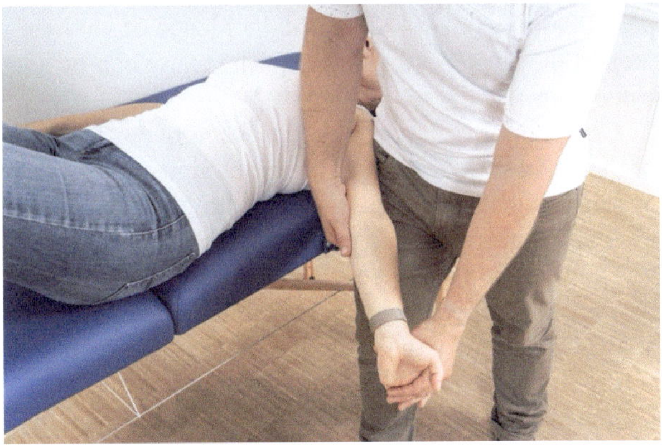

Fig. 18.2 ULNT2A median nerve

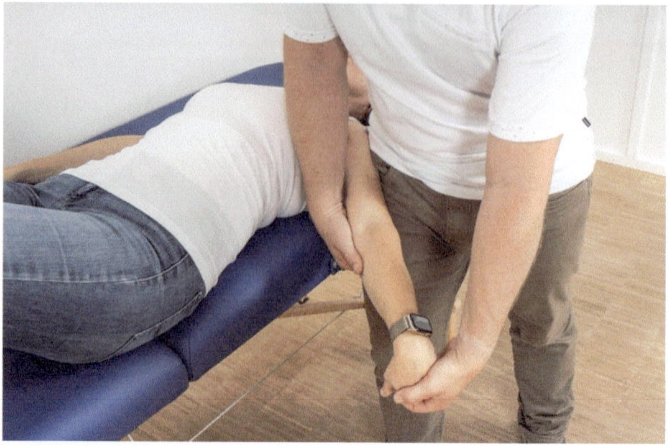

Fig. 18.3 ULNT2B radial nerve

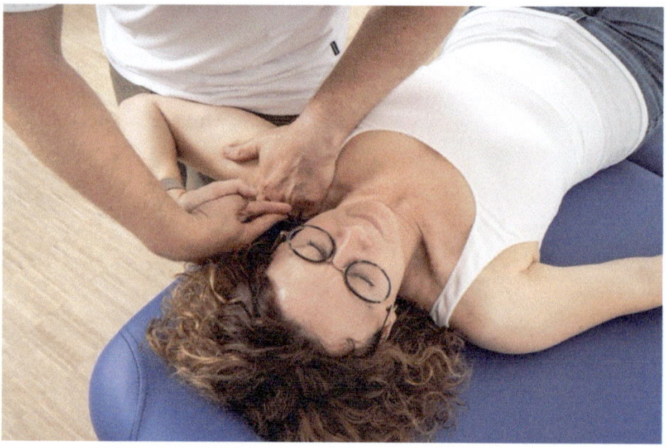

Fig. 18.4 ULNT3 ulnar nerve

What Is Cervical Radiculopathy?

Cervical radiculopathy has an annual incidence of 107.3 per 100,000 men and 63.5 per 100,000 women [271]. The incidence of cervical radiculopathy seems to peak around the ages of 40–50 [272]. The cause can be a herniated disc, spondylosis, or osteophytosis.

Cervical radiculopathy occurs when one or more nerves are affected at the level of the nerve root, resulting in various signs of pain, nerve conduction disorder, such as sensory loss, motor loss, reduced reflexes, or a combination of these. This often involves compression of the cervical nerve roots.

Compression of the cervical nerve root can occur due to protruding disc material or bony osteophytes that exert pressure on the cervical nerve root. Epidemiological studies have shown that the C7 root (C6–C7 herniation) is most commonly affected, followed by the C6 (C5–C6 herniation) and C8 (C7–T1 herniation) nerve roots. Compression of the nerve root by the disc material likely causes nerve damage, both mechanically and chemically. Mechanically, nerve compression can result in local ischemia and nerve damage. However, equally important is the chemical reaction caused by the chronic pressure of nucleus pulposus on the nerve. Disc degeneration and local ischemia activate a pro-inflammatory response, leading to further sensitization and increased pain in the affected area [273].

However, the majority of cases of cervical radiculopathy are caused by cervical spondylosis. Cervical spondylosis refers to degenerative changes that occur in the cervical spine as one ages. In these cases, the breakdown of the disc over the years leads to a decrease in disc height and narrowing of the foramina.

Risk Factors and Prognosis

Risk factors for cervical radiculopathy include smoking, previous lumbar radiculopathy, lifting heavy objects, frequent diving from a diving board, working with vibrating equipment, and playing golf [272, 274, 275]. The course of cervical radiculopathy is favorable in many cases. Almost 90% of patients with cervical radiculopathy were asymptomatic or had only mild symptoms within a 4-year follow-up [271, 276]. Even without treatment, the majority of these patients would have a favorable outcome. There appears to be a favorable natural course with significant improvement within 4–6 months, but the time to full recovery can range from 24 to 36 months. A small portion of those affected may experience residual pain and limitations, but in most cases, full neurological recovery occurs without myelopathy [274].

How Do You Recognize Cervical Radiculopathy?

Cervical radiculopathy can present with a wide range of clinical symptoms, from pain to objective weakness and reduced reflexes. A thorough medical history is an essential first step in diagnosing radiculopathy. Healthcare providers should focus on the location and patterns of pain, tingling, sensory, and motor disturbances. In most cases, cervical radiculopathy can be diagnosed based on history alone [277]. Patients with cervical radiculopathy typically present with unilateral pain, which may radiate to the ipsilateral arm in the corresponding dermatome. However, the absence of arm pain does not rule out the presence of cervical radiculopathy. Additionally, the patient may complain of numbness in the same dermatome, weakness in the corresponding myotome, and/or reduced reflexes [278].

Spurling Neck Compression Test

Provocative tests to aid in the diagnosis of cervical radiculopathy, such as a combination of a positive Spurling test, symptom reduction with cervical axial traction, the shoulder abduction test, Valsalva maneuver, *upper limb tension* tests, and a positive *arm squeeze* test, increase the likelihood of diagnosing cervical radiculopathy

[279, 280]. Spurling's neck compression test is the most commonly used of these techniques and is performed by extending the neck, bending it sideways, and rotating it to the same side, followed by applying downward axial pressure on the head.

The test is considered positive if radicular symptoms radiate into the limb on the same side as where the neck is bent and twisted sideways. The test appears to have high specificity and sensitivity (95% and 92%, respectively) [281]. This test is thought to narrow the neural foramen and reproduce the patient's symptoms.

The cervical axial traction test is performed with the patient in supine, where the examiner applies axial traction to the neck, equivalent to 10–15 kg of force. A reduction in symptoms during traction and an increase or return of symptoms when traction is released are considered a positive outcome, indicating cervical radiculopathy [282].

Shoulder Abduction Test

The shoulder abduction test checks if symptoms decrease when the shoulder is abducted, which reduces the tension on the nerve. The sensitivity of this test ranges from 17% to 78% and the specificity from 75% to 92% [280].

Arm Squeeze Test

The *arm squeeze* test is performed by squeezing the middle third of the patient's upper arm, with the thumb placed on the musculus triceps and the fingers on the biceps brachii muscle. The test is considered positive if the pain is 3 points higher (on a scale of 10) compared to two other areas (the acromioclavicular joint and the subacromial area) [283].

In evaluating cervical radiculopathy, radiographs and advanced imaging techniques, such as CT scans and MRI, are typically used. Radiographs evaluate intervertebral disc height, foramina, and degenerative changes. MRI can also assess soft tissues that may compress nerves and show signs of myelomalacia. Finally, an EMG can be useful to distinguish peripheral nerve entrapment syndromes from cervical radiculopathy.

What Is Hemiplegic Shoulder Pain?

A cerebrovascular accident (CVA) is a common condition worldwide. Due to upper motor neuron damage, a CVA causes a wide range of effects, including changes in muscle tone around the upper limb. Hemiplegic shoulder pain (HSP) is the most common painful condition in patients after a CVA and one of the four most common medical complications post-CVA [284, 285], with a prevalence ranging from 22% to 47% [286]. Incidence rates vary widely, from 16% to 84% [287–290], but a more recent meta-analysis estimates this at 10–22% [286]. The wide variation in HSP prevalence reflects the lack of a clear definition. Unilateral shoulder pain often occurs 2–3 months after a CVA and is a common and disabling complication following a stroke. It can significantly affect the patient's quality of life [291–293].

Typical risk factors for developing HSP include relatively younger age (under 70 years), left-sided hemiparesis, hemorrhagic stroke, medical history, a higher-than-average score (>14/42) on the *National Institutes of Health Stroke Scale*, and the presence of spasticity [286]. And we would almost forget that, in addition to these risk factors, these patients can also develop other shoulder conditions, such as frozen shoulder or RCRSP, or issues with the cervical spine [289].

Other factors likely contributing to HSP include shoulder dislocation [294] or a rotator cuff injury [295]. During recovery after a stroke, it is believed that upper limb spasticity, shoulder dislocation, and limited shoulder joint mobility lead to shoulder pain.

How Do You Recognize Hemiplegic Shoulder Pain?

The clinical presentation of HSP shows reduced shoulder movement on the affected side within the first weeks after a stroke, gradually worsening after 1 month [296–298], along with typical neurological signs such as impaired sensation, hemispatial neglect, spasticity, and flaccid paralysis [299, 300]. Spasticity is one of the characteristic developments, usually occurring between 1 and 6 weeks after a stroke [301]. Spasticity is often defined as a disrupted sensorimotor regulation following an upper motor neuron lesion, manifesting as intermittent or continuous involuntary muscle activity [302]. Clinically, it presents with symptoms such as increased muscle tone (hypertonia), a series of rapid muscle contractions (clonus), muscle spasms, spastic co-contractions, or a combination of these elements [303]. These various clinical manifestations of spasticity make evaluation challenging. This can also cause a lot of pain.

In addition to spasticity, there is often muscle weakness, accompanied by a clear loss of control around the shoulder [304]. This can lead to musculoskeletal issues such as changes in the elasticity of the surrounding muscles. Static contractures may develop, with a combination of increased stiffness and reduced shoulder mobility [305]. The vicious cycle begins with further muscle shortening, leading to an increase in spasticity and pain. In general, we see a pattern of contraction of the shoulder girdle adductors and internal rotators [284, 306], usually accompanied by elbow flexion [307, 308].

What Is Parsonage-Turner Syndrome?

Neuralgic amyotrophy, also known as Parsonage-Turner syndrome (PTS) or brachial neuritis, is a condition of the peripheral nervous system characterized by two prominent features: severe (neuropathic) pain and significant muscle atrophy. PTS is often not immediately recognized, with an average delay of 3–9 months before diagnosis is made. Symptoms have a slow recovery process that can take months to years and often affect the upper extremity. In most cases, a preceding trigger or event can be identified.

In the mid-nineteenth century, two separate conditions were described: paralysis of the musculus serratus anterior muscle and postinfectious paralysis. In 1948, Parsonage and Turner recognized the common characteristics of these conditions and concluded that they were different presentations of the same disorder [309]. They came up with the term "neuralgic amyotrophy" to describe this syndrome, emphasizing its two main clinical features: severe pain and significant muscle loss.

Traditionally, PTS was considered a rare condition, with an estimated annual incidence of 1.64 cases per 100,000 people [310]. However, the actual incidence is much higher, as the condition is often under-recognized. A prospective study reported an incidence of 1 case per 1000 people [311]. PTS typically presents sporadically, usually around the age of 40, and is slightly more common in men. However, there is also a hereditary form, which primarily affects younger individuals around the age of 25 [312]. The latter accounts for approximately 10–19% of PTS cases [312].

How Do You Recognize Parsonage-Turner Syndrome?

PTS primarily manifests with severe neuropathic pain, followed by local paralysis, ranging from isolated paralysis of the anterior interosseous nerve to severe bilateral paralysis of both upper limbs.

Despite this variation, a triad of symptoms is generally recognized. First, the symptoms often begin with a (frequently identifiable) trigger. At least 50% of PTS cases report a trigger, which can include minor trauma, surgery, vaccination, medication use, or even a strenuous physical exertion. But most often these are upper respiratory infections or a flu-like illness, though bacterial infections and other viruses can also cause PTS [313]. The common denominator seems to be the activation of the immune system, which subsequently leads to a selective inflammation of the peripheral nerves. There also often appears to be an underlying predisposition and susceptibility to mechanical injuries of the brachial plexus. Then there is the characteristic pain in the upper limbs and chest area, and, finally, weakness and atrophy become visible. The latter makes diagnosis easier. The neurogenic symptoms are almost always motor in nature. Sensory loss is a less prominent symptom and can often be absent [314, 315].

In 90% of patients, the first symptom is typically pain, which very often (in about 60% of cases) occurs in the middle of the night or is noticed upon waking [312, 316]. The pain increases in intensity over the course of several hours. Due to its severity, it prompts the patient to seek medical attention.

Table 18.1 Clinical presentation of Parsonage-Turner syndrome

Including characteristics	Excluding characteristics
Men with an average age around 40 years	Progressively worsening pain or weakness lasting more than 3 months
Sudden and severe attacks of neuropathic pain in the upper extremity	Only limitations in passive ROM in the glenohumeral joint
Local paresis and atrophy in the muscles around the shoulder	Symmetrical distribution of muscle weakness
After a few days, local motor abnormalities occur, along with atrophy and possibly sensory deficits	
Pain can come on suddenly, such as in the middle of the night while sleeping	
Pain is usually reported laterally at the shoulder and in the musculus trapezius region. Sometimes also in the scapular area, the glenohumeral joint, or distally in the arm	Horner syndrome (neurological condition caused by damage to the sympathetic nerves, resulting in ptosis, miosis, and anhidrosis on the affected side of the face)
Antalgic posture with shoulder adduction and elbow flexion may be present	Head and neck movements influence shoulder-arm pain

The pain is usually localized in one of the arms, most often on the dominant side, although bilateral involvement is also common. The pain is worsened by movements of the shoulder or upper extremity. Interestingly, it is not aggravated by head or neck movements, which distinguishes it from acute radiculopathies. After 1 or 2 weeks, the pain diminishes or is replaced by a dull, aching pain, although some patients report very intense and persistent pain lasting up to about 4 weeks after the onset of symptoms.

Severe pain often masks muscle weakness in the early stages, as patients instinctively avoid shoulder girdle movements. Consequently, any atrophy may go unnoticed for some time. It is only when the pain subsides and the patient begins to move the shoulder that motor deficits and atrophy become more evident, typically taking a few weeks for the atrophy to become visibly noticeable. Additionally, there is no clear relationship with psychological distress [317]. Finally, an EMG can be performed for confirmation (Table 18.1).

19 The Role of Imaging

Imaging can play an important role in the evaluation of patients with shoulder pain, especially when the diagnosis of the pathology is not apparent from clinical examination. It provides healthcare providers with valuable additional information about the anatomical structures of the shoulder, which can assist in diagnosing and planning the appropriate treatment. The imaging techniques we will discuss include X-rays, ultrasound, CT scans, and magnetic resonance imaging (MRI) scans, each with its own advantages and disadvantages. These images can serve as objective information to help make a proper diagnosis.

X-rays and CT images are generated by X-rays passing through the shoulder. However, X-rays are a form of ionizing radiation, and it is suspected that they may increase the risk of cancer, though this effect on the already high-risk figures does not appear to be significant [318]. The radiation dose from an X-ray is very low (0.01 mSv), but that of a CT scan can reach 2.8 mSv. This is roughly the equivalent to the annual natural radiation from the sun and earth. Therefore, caution is especially required with the latter.

Ultrasound and MRI are techniques that do not use ionizing radiation and are therefore not subject to these risks. However, they also have disadvantages. The strong magnetic field of an MRI, for example, can cause metal objects inside or on the patient to move or heat up during the scan. It is important that the referring physician notes this when making the referral and the patient is rescreened before entering the scanner. Newer surgical prostheses (such as joint prostheses) are now MRI compatible. The biggest drawback now is that they cause artifacts that can obscure the area being scanned.

However, it is important to note that imaging is not always necessary for every patient with shoulder pain. It must be carefully considered and supplemented with a thorough clinical evaluation, including listening to the patient's story. As previously discussed, there is a poor correlation between pain and structural pathology (such as rotator cuff tears) [155]. Moreover, imaging findings rarely influence non-surgical management. Also, imaging findings can hinder patient involvement and increase anxiety and avoidance behavior [154].

F. Struyf, *Shoulder Pain*, https://doi.org/10.1007/978-3-031-82228-5_19

Rotator Cuff-Related Shoulder Pain (RCRSP)

Imaging may be required to rule out tumors, fractures, dislocations, or other red flags. An X-ray can be used to exclude glenohumeral osteoarthritis or calcific tendinopathy. Ultrasound imaging, on the other hand, can be useful to objectify subacromial bursitis, partial or complete tears, calcifications, or degenerative changes around the AC and/or glenohumeral joint.

MRI can also be an excellent imaging technique for observing similar abnormalities as ultrasound but only statically. While ultrasound imaging is likely the best option for detecting calcifications in tendons, MRI is better at registering articular, bony, and muscular pathologies.

CT scans generally do not offer much additional value compared to the aforementioned imaging techniques, except perhaps for visualizing rarer bone pathologies. In RCRSP patients who are following the expected improvement trajectory, imaging is usually not necessary, and it is only applicable for differential diagnosis.

Biceps Tendon Disorders

Long head biceps tendon (LHBT) tendinopathy is difficult to identify through imaging. There is still debate about the use of imaging in diagnosing LHBT tendinopathies. When a partial or complete rupture of the LHBT is suspected, the diagnostic value of imaging increases significantly. Generally, ultrasound imaging reports high specificity for detecting dislocations (76% sensitivity and 98% specificity), partial tears (sensitivity ranging from 27% to 100% and 100% specificity), and complete ruptures (71% sensitivity and 98% specificity). Overall, the results indicate fairly high specificity, but sensitivity shows more variation [167].

The use of X-rays is less obvious when it comes to imaging soft tissues. However, X-rays are sometimes used to visualize bony abnormalities in the bicipital groove. Generally, the diagnostic accuracy, specificity, and sensitivity of *magnetic resonance arthrography* (MRA) are slightly better than MRI, but both showed variability in diagnosing LHB tendinopathy.

Labral Injuries

Diagnosing labral injuries based solely on clinical examination is difficult. Additional imaging techniques such as X-rays, CT scans, and MR arthrography can be used. Currently, CT arthrography is the most commonly used imaging technique, with a sensitivity of 94–98% and a specificity of 73–88% [319]. However, MRI and MR arthrography are considered the gold standard. The sensitivity and specificity of MR arthrography range between 82–89% and 91–98%, respectively. If there is suspicion of an associated bone injury, CT arthrography may have advantages over MR arthrography.

A Rotator Cuff Tear

Imaging can be helpful in determining the size and location of rotator cuff tears. *Magnetic resonance imaging* (MRI) is usually the best method to visualize the exact location of the tear. Additionally, MRI can assess muscle quality, which is relevant for the decision regarding surgery. Ultrasound imaging, MRI, and MRA have similar positive and negative likelihood ratios for diagnosing partial-thickness tears (LR+ = approx. 11; LR− = approx. 0.3) [320]. For full-thickness tears, this increases to an LR+ of around 13 for ultrasound imaging and MRI and an LR− of 0.1 for ultrasound imaging, MRI, and MRA. The LR+ for MRA is even 18.

Calcific Tendinopathy

To diagnose calcific tendinopathy and objectively confirm the presence of calcifications, imaging is necessary. Due to its ability to visualize calcifications without radiation and detect neovascularization, ultrasound imaging appears to be the preferred method [321–323]. Indeed, ultrasound imaging is a valid and practical imaging technique for diagnosing calcific tendinopathy. In addition to ultrasound, standard X-rays can be used to visualize calcifications in the supraspinatus tendon. Other imaging options, such as MRI, can also be considered. Although the presence or absence of calcification can be determined, the clinical significance of these deposits remains uncertain.

Frozen Shoulder

In practice, a working diagnosis can often be made based on a thorough patient history and clinical examination, without necessarily needing imaging in primary healthcare [324].

However, standard X-rays of the glenohumeral joint are often recommended for differential diagnosis. This is to ensure that there are no substantial degenerative joint changes that could also cause pain and restricted movement, such as osteoarthritis. Additionally, a posterior dislocation can present a similar clinical picture, though a trauma would typically be reported in the patient's history. Rare humeral bone tumors can also be ruled out this way.

The use of advanced imaging modalities, such as MRI, has also been suggested for diagnosing frozen shoulder. Findings such as thickening of the axillary capsule and/or obliteration of the axillary recess, thickening of the coracohumeral ligament and the rotator interval, and/or hypervascularity are considered indicative of a frozen shoulder when the imaging results match the clinical presentation [325, 326].

Although soft tissue tumors are only present in less than 1% of patients with frozen shoulder, advanced imaging may be of great importance for those with persistent symptoms [327]. However, routine use of advanced imaging is not recommended, as it does not provide superior diagnostic information beyond history taking and physical examination [328].

The role of ultrasound imaging in patients suspected of having a frozen shoulder is primarily in guiding subacromial and intra-articular injections or hydrodilatation.

Glenohumeral Instability

In cases of traumatic dislocations, an X-ray can clearly show an anterior or posterior dislocated glenohumeral joint. However, it is important that these images are not only taken in a frontal plane. In a frontal view, the joint may appear normal if the humeral head is aligned with the glenoid. Other angles (such as axillary views) are just as important to avoid missing dislocations. A simple X-ray can also provide an image of any possible bony Bankart or Hill-Sachs lesion. For labral injuries, MRI and MR arthrography are considered the gold standard. On the other hand, functional glenohumeral instability is usually diagnosed clinically and often does not require imaging.

Acromioclavicular, Sternoclavicular, and Clavicular Conditions

The original Rockwood classification is based on X-ray findings, although the reliability is variable and often only moderate [329, 330]. However, radiographic imaging is usually necessary to rule out clavicle fractures in both AC and SC injuries.

Computed tomography does not significantly improve reliability [329]. In contrast, ultrasound imaging has been shown to achieve a high degree of sensitivity (80%) and specificity (100%), especially for detecting detachment of the deltoid and trapezius muscles [331]. Ultrasound imaging can also be used to support the diagnostic and therapeutic effects of corticosteroid injections [247]. Lastly, MRI can be used to better visualize soft tissue injuries. MRI is especially helpful in supporting the decision of whether surgery is necessary [332, 333].

Glenohumeral Osteoarthritis

Clear X-rays of the shoulder are essential to confirm the diagnosis. Anteroposterior, lateral, and axillary views are recommended. The radiological definitions of osteoarthritis rely on identifying radiographic features of joint damage. However, many different radiographic classification systems have been described.

Radiographic changes include joint space narrowing, osteophyte formation, periarticular cysts, cranial migration of the humeral head, and subchondral sclerosis. It is clear that combining the patient's symptoms with anatomically proven joint damage leads to the most accurate diagnosis. But again, keep in mind that radiological signs of damage can also be present in asymptomatic individuals [254, 334, 335]. Therefore, it is not recommended to diagnose a patient based solely on imaging.

In addition to X-rays, CT arthrography can also be used. This technique allows for the creation of a 3D image, which can provide a detailed view of glenoid morphology or bone density and is recommended when considering a shoulder prosthesis.

For soft tissue imaging, MRI is superior. However, MRI is not routinely recommended for diagnosing glenohumeral osteoarthritis, though it may be useful for a subset of patients with unclear diagnoses or suspected peri-articular tumors.

Communication with the Patient 20

We all understand the importance of communication, but even those who feel they excel at it should continue to reflect on their skills. Perfect communication is an illusion, and there is no one-size-fits-all approach. We all make mistakes and seek to improve. Hopefully, this chapter will provide some valuable insights.

The first priority is to avoid exacerbating the fear that many of your patients already feel. Our messages can sometimes unintentionally heighten their anxiety, which can make them more vulnerable and less self-reliant, outcomes we want to prevent. The language we use in clinical practice holds significant power. It can offer support but can also lead to lasting harm. The words we choose can shape how others think, feel, and act, ultimately affecting the clinical outcome.

Let us begin at the start. A patient arrives with a problem and describes it in their own words. However, patients often struggle to articulate their complaints clearly, relying on metaphors to give shape to their emotions. Pain can feel chaotic, and metaphors help impose some order in that chaos. Each person's experience of pain is unique and much like exploring a new galaxy through a telescope; through communication, we strive to understand the patient's perspective.

It is important to remember that our patients do not always think like we do. They come from diverse backgrounds, with different beliefs, experiences, cultures, and vocabularies. Their world often differs significantly from ours. Despite these differences, we must make an effort to understand their experiences through our conversations. When discussing our findings, we need to be mindful of our language. Our terminology may be unfamiliar or even interpreted negatively by the patient. Our words can have lasting consequences; they can offer warmth and clarity, but they can also cause harm.

F. Struyf, *Shoulder Pain*, https://doi.org/10.1007/978-3-031-82228-5_20

Validating Versus Reassurance

Pain and its associated effects, like anxiety, are often invisible and can be described vaguely in a patient's history. To truly recognize this anxiety, we need to learn how to listen. Try to put yourself in the patient's shoes to better understand their perspectives and experiences. This practice can help you become attuned to the unspoken cries for help and validate their struggles. Additionally, give your full attention when others speak. Ask open-ended questions and encourage them to express themselves freely.

And when listening, make sure the person knows that we have heard it. It is a good start to look the patient in the eye and nod in affirmation, but this is often not enough. It is also about the follow-up questions you ask. If you let your patient speak for a few minutes without interruption and then focus on an element that does not touch on the core issue (such as the patient's suffering), the patient may repeat part of their story or become frustrated, feeling they have not been truly heard.

Pay close attention to the patient's body language as well. Are they showing signs of resistance? It may be that your patient does not feel heard. It is not easy. A good way to reduce a patient's anxiety is through validating. Validating means telling that the patient's story is understandable and accepting it as a reasonable possibility [336]. We may be excellent at our jobs and show empathy with family and friends, but we often fail to show it enough to the patient. The belief that an empathic response (such as validating pain) would only reinforce pain behavior has already been dismissed as unproven [336]. Validating could just as easily translate into increased trust in the clinician, making the patient feel better and reducing their pain behavior [336]. The future will provide more clarity on this.

However, validating is not the same as reassurance. Reassurance involves giving optimistic messages to patients, like "You don't need to worry. We are experienced and have treated this condition many times. Everything will be fine." These kinds of vague promises will not convince all patients and can instead lead to anxiety and negative feelings.

Listening as Therapy

This book focuses on the evaluation of shoulder complaints, not on their treatment. However, I cannot resist offering a small suggestion that could already benefit your patients. It turns out that during your history taking and clinical examination, you can already have an impact on the final outcome. Your assessment is also the beginning of your therapy. Everyone can probably recall a moment when the very first consultation had a significant effect on the patient's symptoms. Patients may even offer an explanation for this effect: "I feel better now that we've talked about my complaint and now that we have a plan."

We are often quick to assume that what you said influenced the patient's understanding of their illness or beliefs. And that may be true, but do not underestimate the power of simply listening and acknowledging the patient. The key is not always in how much information you provided, and it may not even be the quality of the information you shared. The connection you established with your patient may have been the key factor. And it is precisely your communication and your attentive listening that can have a significant impact on the relationship with your patient.

► The most important thing to remember can be illustrated with a metaphor: When the conductor overshadows the orchestra, something is wrong. True harmony in communication occurs when we, as clinicians, create space for our patients' melodies to be heard.

References

1. Roach NT, Venkadesan M, Rainbow MJ, Lieberman DE. Elastic energy storage in the shoulder and the evolution of high-speed throwing in Homo. Nature. 2013;498(7455):483–6.
2. Hill CL, Gill TK, Shanahan EM, Taylor AW. Prevalence and correlates of shoulder pain and stiffness in a population-based study: the North West Adelaide Health Study. Int J Rheum Dis. 2010;13(3):215–22.
3. Urwin M, Symmons D, Allison T, Brammah T, Busby H, Roxby M, et al. Estimating the burden of musculoskeletal disorders in the community: the comparative prevalence of symptoms at different anatomical sites, and the relation to social deprivation. Ann Rheum Dis. 1998;57(11):649–55.
4. Linsell L, Dawson J, Zondervan K, Rose P, Randall T, Fitzpatrick R, et al. Prevalence and incidence of adults consulting for shoulder conditions in UK primary care; patterns of diagnosis and referral. Rheumatology (Oxford). 2006;45(2):215–21.
5. Luime JJ, Koes BW, Hendriksen IJ, Burdorf A, Verhagen AP, Miedema HS, et al. Prevalence and incidence of shoulder pain in the general population; a systematic review. Scand J Rheumatol. 2004;33(2):73–81.
6. Harkness EF, Macfarlane GJ, Nahit ES, Silman AJ, McBeth J. Mechanical and psychosocial factors predict new onset shoulder pain: a prospective cohort study of newly employed workers. Occup Environ Med. 2003;60(11):850–7.
7. van der Windt DA, Thomas E, Pope DP, de Winter AF, Macfarlane GJ, Bouter LM, et al. Occupational risk factors for shoulder pain: a systematic review. Occup Environ Med. 2000;57(7):433–42.
8. van der Windt DA, Koes BW, Boeke AJ, Deville W, De Jong BA, Bouter LM. Shoulder disorders in general practice: prognostic indicators of outcome. Br J Gen Pract. 1996;46(410):519–23.
9. Virta L, Joranger P, Brox JI, Eriksson R. Costs of shoulder pain and resource use in primary health care: a cost-of-illness study in Sweden. BMC Musculoskelet Disord. 2012;13:17.
10. Kuijpers T, van Tulder MW, van der Heijden GJ, Bouter LM, van der Windt DA. Costs of shoulder pain in primary care consulters: a prospective cohort study in The Netherlands. BMC Musculoskelet Disord. 2006;7:83.
11. Marks D, Comans T, Bisset L, Thomas M, Scuffham PA. Shoulder pain cost-of-illness in patients referred for public orthopaedic care in Australia. Aust Health Rev. 2019;43(5):540–8.
12. Soslowsky LJ, Flatow EL, Bigliani LU, Pawluk RJ, Ateshian GA, Mow VC. Quantitation of in situ contact areas at the glenohumeral joint: a biomechanical study. J Orthop Res. 1992;10(4):524–34.
13. Howell SM, Galinat BJ. The glenoid-labral socket. A constrained articular surface. Clin Orthop Relat Res. 1989;243:122–5.
14. Witherspoon JW, Smirnova IV, McIff TE. Neuroanatomical distribution of mechanoreceptors in the human cadaveric shoulder capsule and labrum. J Anat. 2014;225(3):337–45.
15. Hertel R, Knothe U, Ballmer FT. Geometry of the proximal humerus and implications for prosthetic design. J Shoulder Elbow Surg. 2002;11(4):331–8.

F. Struyf, *Shoulder Pain*, https://doi.org/10.1007/978-3-031-82228-5

16. Huri G, Kaymakoglu M, Garbis N. Rotator cable and rotator interval: anatomy, biomechanics and clinical importance. EFORT Open Rev. 2019;4(2):56–62.
17. Clark J, Sidles JA, Matsen FA. The relationship of the glenohumeral joint capsule to the rotator cuff. Clin Orthop Relat Res. 1990;254:29–34.
18. Clark JM, Harryman DT 2nd. Tendons, ligaments, and capsule of the rotator cuff. Gross and microscopic anatomy. J Bone Joint Surg Am. 1992;74(5):713–25.
19. ElMaraghy AW, Devereaux MW. A systematic review and comprehensive classification of pectoralis major tears. J Shoulder Elbow Surg. 2012;21(3):412–22.
20. Ludewig PM, Behrens SA, Meyer SM, Spoden SM, Wilson LA. Three-dimensional clavicular motion during arm elevation: reliability and descriptive data. J Orthop Sports Phys Ther. 2004;34(3):140–9.
21. McClure PW, Michener LA, Karduna AR. Shoulder function and 3-dimensional scapular kinematics in people with and without shoulder impingement syndrome. Phys Ther. 2006;86(8):1075–90.
22. Ludewig PM, Phadke V, Braman JP, Hassett DR, Cieminski CJ, LaPrade RF. Motion of the shoulder complex during multiplanar humeral elevation. J Bone Joint Surg Am. 2009;91(2):378–89.
23. Struyf F, Nijs J, Baeyens J-P, Mottram S, Meeusen R. Scapular positioning and movement in unimpaired shoulders, shoulder impingement syndrome, and glenohumeral instability. Scand J Med Sci Sports. 2011;21(3):352–8.
24. Landin D, Thompson M, Jackson MR. Actions of the biceps Brachii at the shoulder: a review. J Clin Med Res. 2017;9(8):667–70.
25. Martin C, Bideau B, Bideau N, Nicolas G, Delamarche P, Kulpa R. Energy flow analysis during the tennis serve: comparison between injured and noninjured tennis players. Am J Sports Med. 2014;42(11):2751–60.
26. Chu SK, Jayabalan P, Kibler WB, Press J. The Kinetic Chain revisited: new concepts on throwing mechanics and injury. PM R. 2016;8(3 Suppl):S69–77.
27. Endo Y, Sakamoto M. Correlation of shoulder and elbow injuries with muscle tightness, core stability, and balance by longitudinal measurements in junior high school baseball players. J Phys Ther Sci. 2014;26(5):689–93.
28. Laudner K, Wong R, Onuki T, Lynall R, Meister K. The relationship between clinically measured hip rotational motion and shoulder biomechanics during the pitching motion. J Sci Med Sport. 2015;18(5):581–4.
29. Robb AJ, Fleisig G, Wilk K, Macrina L, Bolt B, Pajaczkowski J. Passive ranges of motion of the hips and their relationship with pitching biomechanics and ball velocity in professional baseball pitchers. Am J Sports Med. 2010;38(12):2487–93.
30. Scher S, Anderson K, Weber N, Bajorek J, Rand K, Bey MJ. Associations among hip and shoulder range of motion and shoulder injury in professional baseball players. J Athl Train. 2010;45(2):191–7.
31. Lintner D, Noonan TJ, Kibler WB. Injury patterns and biomechanics of the athlete's shoulder. Clin Sports Med. 2008;27(4):527–51.
32. Roy JS, MacDermid JC, Woodhouse LJ. Measuring shoulder function: a systematic review of four questionnaires. Arthritis Rheum. 2009;61(5):623–32.
33. Dabija DI, Jain NB. Minimal clinically important difference of shoulder outcome measures and diagnoses: a systematic review. Am J Phys Med Rehabil. 2019;98(8):671–6.
34. Bull C, Byrnes J, Hettiarachchi R, Downes M. A systematic review of the validity and reliability of patient-reported experience measures. Health Serv Res. 2019;54(5):1023–35.
35. Lyne SA, Goldblatt FM, Shanahan EM. Living with a frozen shoulder—a phenomenological inquiry. BMC Musculoskelet Disord. 2022;23(1):318.
36. Harding G, Parsons S, Rahman A, Underwood M. "It struck me that they didn't understand pain": the specialist pain clinic experience of patients with chronic musculoskeletal pain. Arthritis Rheum. 2005;53(5):691–6.
37. Tashjian RZ, Deloach J, Porucznik CA, Powell AP. Minimal clinically important differences (MCID) and patient acceptable symptomatic state (PASS) for visual analog scales

(VAS) measuring pain in patients treated for rotator cuff disease. J Shoulder Elbow Surg. 2009;18(6):927–32.
38. Mintken PE, Glynn P, Cleland JA. Psychometric properties of the shortened disabilities of the Arm, Shoulder, and Hand Questionnaire (QuickDASH) and Numeric Pain Rating Scale in patients with shoulder pain. J Shoulder Elbow Surg. 2009;18(6):920–6.
39. Mease PJ, Spaeth M, Clauw DJ, Arnold LM, Bradley LA, Russell IJ, et al. Estimation of minimum clinically important difference for pain in fibromyalgia. Arthritis Care Res (Hoboken). 2011;63(6):821–6.
40. Roy JS, MacDermid JC, Woodhouse LJ. A systematic review of the psychometric properties of the Constant-Murley score. J Shoulder Elbow Surg. 2010;19(1):157–64.
41. Angst F, Schwyzer HK, Aeschlimann A, Simmen BR, Goldhahn J. Measures of adult shoulder function: disabilities of the Arm, Shoulder, and Hand Questionnaire (DASH) and its short version (QuickDASH), Shoulder Pain and Disability Index (SPADI), American Shoulder and Elbow Surgeons (ASES) Society standardized shoulder assessment form, Constant (Murley) Score (CS), Simple Shoulder Test (SST), Oxford Shoulder Score (OSS), Shoulder Disability Questionnaire (SDQ), and Western Ontario Shoulder Instability Index (WOSI). Arthritis Care Res (Hoboken). 2011;63(Suppl 11):S174–88.
42. Thoomes-de Graaf M, Scholten-Peeters W, Duijn E, Karel Y, de Vet HC, Koes B, et al. The responsiveness and interpretability of the shoulder pain and disability index. J Orthop Sports Phys Ther. 2017;47(4):278–86.
43. van Kampen DA, Willems WJ, van Beers LW, Castelein RM, Scholtes VA, Terwee CB. Determination and comparison of the smallest detectable change (SDC) and the minimal important change (MIC) of four-shoulder patient-reported outcome measures (PROMs). J Orthop Surg Res. 2013;8:40.
44. MacDermid JC, Drosdowech D, Faber K. Responsiveness of self-report scales in patients recovering from rotator cuff surgery. J Shoulder Elbow Surg. 2006;15(4):407–14.
45. Braun C, Handoll HH. Estimating the minimal important difference for the Western Ontario Rotator Cuff Index (WORC) in adults with shoulder pain associated with partial-thickness rotator cuff tears. Musculoskelet Sci Pract. 2018;35:30–3.
46. Kennedy CA, Beaton DE. A user's survey of the clinical application and content validity of the DASH (Disabilities of the Arm, Shoulder and Hand) outcome measure. J Hand Ther. 2017;30(1):30–40 e2.
47. Gabel CP, Michener LA, Burkett B, Neller A. The Upper Limb Functional Index: development and determination of reliability, validity, and responsiveness. J Hand Ther. 2006;19(3):328–48; quiz 49.
48. Schmitt JS, Di Fabio RP. Reliable change and minimum important difference (MID) proportions facilitated group responsiveness comparisons using individual threshold criteria. J Clin Epidemiol. 2004;57(10):1008–18.
49. van der Linde JA, Willems WJ, van Kampen DA, van Beers LW, van Deurzen DF, Terwee CB. Measurement properties of the Western Ontario Shoulder Instability index in Dutch patients with shoulder instability. BMC Musculoskelet Disord. 2014;15:211.
50. Whittle JH, Peters SE, Manzanero S, Duke PF. A systematic review of patient-reported outcome measures used in shoulder instability research. J Shoulder Elbow Surg. 2020;29(2):381–91.
51. Foong WS, Zeng GJ, Goh GS, Hao Y, Lie DTT, Chang PCC. Determining the minimal clinically important difference on the Oxford shoulder instability score in patients undergoing arthroscopic Bankart repair for shoulder instability. Orthop J Sports Med. 2022;10(1):23259671211060023.
52. Demir Y, Sjoberg H, Stark A, Salomonsson B. Western Ontario Osteoarthritis of the Shoulder Index (WOOS)—a validation for use in proximal humerus fractures treated with arthroplasty. BMC Musculoskelet Disord. 2023;24(1):450.
53. Hallberg K, Salomonsson B. Validity, reliability, and responsiveness of the Swedish version of Western Ontario Osteoarthritis of the Shoulder index. BMC Musculoskelet Disord. 2022;23(1):351.

54. Ozal S, Atalay Guzel N, Kaptan AY, Eren TK, Kafa N. Validity and reliability of the turkish version of Western Ontario Osteoarthritis of the Shoulder Index. Jt Dis Relat Surg. 2021;32(2):497–503.
55. Corona K, Cerciello S, Morris BJ, Visona E, Merolla G, Porcellini G. Cross-cultural adaptation and validation of the Italian version of the Western Ontario Osteoarthritis of the Shoulder index (WOOS). J Orthop Traumatol. 2016;17(4):309–13.
56. Lo IK, Griffin S, Kirkley A. The development of a disease-specific quality of life measurement tool for osteoarthritis of the shoulder: the Western Ontario Osteoarthritis of the Shoulder (WOOS) index. Osteoarthritis Cartilage. 2001;9(8):771–8.
57. Nyring MRK, Olsen BS, Amundsen A, Rasmussen JV. Minimal Clinically Important Differences (MCID) for the Western Ontario Osteoarthritis of the Shoulder Index (WOOS) and the Oxford Shoulder Score (OSS). Patient Relat Outcome Meas. 2021;12:299–306.
58. Jones IA, Togashi R, Heckmann N, Vangsness CT Jr. Minimal clinically important difference (MCID) for patient-reported shoulder outcomes. J Shoulder Elbow Surg. 2020;29(7):1484–92.
59. Richards RR, An KN, Bigliani LU, Friedman RJ, Gartsman GM, Gristina AG, et al. A standardized method for the assessment of shoulder function. J Shoulder Elbow Surg. 1994;3(6):347–52.
60. Mintken PE, Cleland JA, Whitman JM, George SZ. Psychometric properties of the fear-avoidance beliefs questionnaire and Tampa scale of kinesiophobia in patients with shoulder pain. Arch Phys Med Rehabil. 2010;91(7):1128–36.
61. Miller R, Todd SD. The Tampa scale: a measure of kinesiophobia. Clin J Pain. 1991;7(1):51–2.
62. Sullivan MJ, Bishop SR, Pivik J. The pain catastrophizing scale: development and validation. Psychol Assess. 1995;7(4):524.
63. Grobet C, Marks M, Tecklenburg L, Audige L. Application and measurement properties of EQ-5D to measure quality of life in patients with upper extremity orthopaedic disorders: a systematic literature review. Arch Orthop Trauma Surg. 2018;138(7):953–61.
64. Greenhalgh S, Finucane LM, Mercer C, Selfe J. Safety netting; best practice in the face of uncertainty. Musculoskelet Sci Pract. 2020;48:102179.
65. McClure PW, Michener LA. Staged approach for rehabilitation classification: shoulder disorders (STAR-shoulder). Phys Ther. 2015;95(5):791–800.
66. Dejaco C, Brouwer E, Mason JC, Buttgereit F, Matteson EL, Dasgupta B. Giant cell arteritis and polymyalgia rheumatica: current challenges and opportunities. Nat Rev Rheumatol. 2017;13(10):578–92.
67. Rosenthal AK, Ryan LM. Calcium pyrophosphate deposition disease. N Engl J Med. 2016;374(26):2575–84.
68. Swarup I, Henn CM, Nguyen JT, Dines DM, Craig EV, Warren RF, et al. Effect of pre-operative expectations on the outcomes following total shoulder arthroplasty. Bone Joint J. 2017;99-B(9):1190–6.
69. Bullington J, Nordemar R, Nordemar K, Sjostrom-Flanagan C. Meaning out of chaos: a way to understand chronic pain. Scand J Caring Sci. 2003;17(4):325–31.
70. Chester R, Jerosch-Herold C, Lewis J, Shepstone L. Psychological factors are associated with the outcome of physiotherapy for people with shoulder pain: a multicentre longitudinal cohort study. Br J Sports Med. 2018;52(4):269–75.
71. De Baets L, Matheve T, Meeus M, Struyf F, Timmermans A. The influence of cognitions, emotions and behavioral factors on treatment outcomes in musculoskeletal shoulder pain: a systematic review. Clin Rehabil. 2019;33(6):980–91.
72. Martinez-Calderon J, Meeus M, Struyf F, Diaz-Cerrillo JL, Clavero-Cano S, Morales-Asencio JM, et al. Psychological factors are associated with local and generalized pressure pain hypersensitivity, pain intensity, and function in people with chronic shoulder pain: a cross-sectional study. Musculoskelet Sci Pract. 2019;44:102064.
73. Martinez-Calderon J, Meeus M, Struyf F, Miguel Morales-Asencio J, Gijon-Nogueron G, Luque-Suarez A. The role of psychological factors in the perpetuation of pain intensity and disability in people with chronic shoulder pain: a systematic review. BMJ Open. 2018;8(4):e020703.

74. Reilingh ML, Kuijpers T, Tanja-Harfterkamp AM, van der Windt DA. Course and prognosis of shoulder symptoms in general practice. Rheumatology (Oxford). 2008;47(5):724–30.
75. Struyf F, Geraets J, Noten S, Meeus M, Nijs J. A multivariable prediction model for the chronification of non-traumatic shoulder pain: a systematic review. Pain Physician. 2016;19(2):1–10.
76. Gill TK, Shanahan EM, Taylor AW, Buchbinder R, Hill CL. Shoulder pain in the community: an examination of associative factors using a longitudinal cohort study. Arthritis Care Res (Hoboken). 2013;65(12):2000–7.
77. Applegate KA, Thiese MS, Merryweather AS, Kapellusch J, Drury DL, Wood E, et al. Association between cardiovascular disease risk factors and rotator cuff tendinopathy: a cross-sectional study. J Occup Environ Med. 2017;59(2):154–60.
78. Anisman H, Merali Z, Hayley S. Neurotransmitter, peptide and cytokine processes in relation to depressive disorder: comorbidity between depression and neurodegenerative disorders. Prog Neurobiol. 2008;85(1):1–74.
79. Valkanova V, Ebmeier KP, Allan CL. CRP, IL-6 and depression: a systematic review and meta-analysis of longitudinal studies. J Affect Disord. 2013;150(3):736–44.
80. Capuron L, Lasselin J, Castanon N. Role of adiposity-driven inflammation in depressive morbidity. Neuropsychopharmacology. 2017;42(1):115–28.
81. Gardner T, Refshauge K, Smith L, McAuley J, Hubscher M, Goodall S. Physiotherapists' beliefs and attitudes influence clinical practice in chronic low back pain: a systematic review of quantitative and qualitative studies. J Physiother. 2017;63(3):132–43.
82. Darlow B, Fullen BM, Dean S, Hurley DA, Baxter GD, Dowell A. The association between health care professional attitudes and beliefs and the attitudes and beliefs, clinical management, and outcomes of patients with low back pain: a systematic review. Eur J Pain. 2012;16(1):3–17.
83. Molsted S, Tribler J, Snorgaard O. Musculoskeletal pain in patients with type 2 diabetes. Diabetes Res Clin Pract. 2012;96(2):135–40.
84. Cole A, Gill TK, Shanahan EM, Phillips P, Taylor AW, Hill CL. Is diabetes associated with shoulder pain or stiffness? Results from a population based study. J Rheumatol. 2009;36(2):371–7.
85. Kiani J, Goharifar H, Moghimbeigi A, Azizkhani H. Prevalence and risk factors of five most common upper extremity disorders in diabetics. J Res Health Sci. 2014;14(1):92–5.
86. Polli A, Ickmans K, Godderis L, Nijs J. When environment meets genetics: a clinical review of the epigenetics of pain, psychological factors, and physical activity. Arch Phys Med Rehabil. 2019;100(6):1153–61.
87. Fessel G, Li Y, Diederich V, Guizar-Sicairos M, Schneider P, Sell DR, et al. Advanced glycation end-products reduce collagen molecular sliding to affect collagen fibril damage mechanisms but not stiffness. PLoS One. 2014;9(11):e110948.
88. Struyf F, Mertens MG, Navarro-Ledesma S. Causes of shoulder dysfunction in diabetic patients: a review of literature. Int J Environ Res Public Health. 2022;19(10):6228.
89. Voloshin I, Gelinas J, Maloney MD, O'Keefe RJ, Bigliani LU, Blaine TA. Proinflammatory cytokines and metalloproteases are expressed in the subacromial bursa in patients with rotator cuff disease. Arthroscopy. 2005;21(9):1076e1–9.
90. Dean E, Gormsen Hansen R. Prescribing optimal nutrition and physical activity as "first-line" interventions for best practice management of chronic low-grade inflammation associated with osteoarthritis: evidence synthesis. Arthritis. 2012;2012:560634.
91. Henson J, Yates T, Edwardson CL, Khunti K, Talbot D, Gray LJ, et al. Sedentary time and markers of chronic low-grade inflammation in a high risk population. PLoS One. 2013;8(10):e78350.
92. Strzelak A, Ratajczak A, Adamiec A, Feleszko W. Tobacco smoke induces and alters immune responses in the lung triggering inflammation, allergy, asthma and other lung diseases: a mechanistic review. Int J Environ Res Public Health. 2018;15(5):1033.
93. Sopori M. Effects of cigarette smoke on the immune system. Nat Rev Immunol. 2002;2(5):372–7.

94. Bishop JY, Santiago-Torres JE, Rimmke N, Flanigan DC. Smoking predisposes to rotator cuff pathology and shoulder dysfunction: a systematic review. Arthroscopy. 2015;31(8):1598–605.
95. Millar NL, Reilly JH, Kerr SC, Campbell AL, Little KJ, Leach WJ, et al. Hypoxia: a critical regulator of early human tendinopathy. Ann Rheum Dis. 2012;71(2):302–10.
96. Lundgreen K, Lian OB, Scott A, Nassab P, Fearon A, Engebretsen L. Rotator cuff tear degeneration and cell apoptosis in smokers versus nonsmokers. Arthroscopy. 2014;30(8):936–41.
97. Gillespie MA, Cznik AM, Wassinger CA, Sole G. Rotator cuff-related pain: patients' understanding and experiences. Musculoskelet Sci Pract. 2017;30:64–71.
98. Haack M, Sanchez E, Mullington JM. Elevated inflammatory markers in response to prolonged sleep restriction are associated with increased pain experience in healthy volunteers. Sleep. 2007;30(9):1145–52.
99. Irwin MR, Carrillo C, Olmstead R. Sleep loss activates cellular markers of inflammation: sex differences. Brain Behav Immun. 2010;24(1):54–7.
100. Longo UG, Facchinetti G, Marchetti A, Candela V, Risi Ambrogioni L, Faldetta A, et al. Sleep disturbance and rotator cuff tears: a systematic review. Medicina (Kaunas). 2019;55(8):453.
101. Afolalu EF, Ramlee F, Tang NKY. Effects of sleep changes on pain-related health outcomes in the general population: a systematic review of longitudinal studies with exploratory meta-analysis. Sleep Med Rev. 2018;39:82–97.
102. Kolber MJ, Hanney WJ. The reliability and concurrent validity of shoulder mobility measurements using a digital inclinometer and goniometer: a technical report. Int J Sports Phys Ther. 2012;7(3):306–13.
103. Hayes K, Walton JR, Szomor ZL, Murrell GA. Reliability of 3 methods for assessing shoulder strength. J Shoulder Elbow Surg. 2002;11(1):33–9.
104. Sapega AA. Muscle performance evaluation in orthopaedic practice. J Bone Joint Surg Am. 1990;72(10):1562–74.
105. Wadsworth CT, Krishnan R, Sear M, Harrold J, Nielsen DH. Intrarater reliability of manual muscle testing and hand-held dynametric muscle testing. Phys Ther. 1987;67(9):1342–7.
106. Oh JH, Yoon JP, Kim JY, Oh CH. Isokinetic muscle performance test can predict the status of rotator cuff muscle. Clin Orthop Relat Res. 2010;468(6):1506–13.
107. Itoi E, Minagawa H, Sato T, Sato K, Tabata S. Isokinetic strength after tears of the supraspinatus tendon. J Bone Joint Surg Br. 1997;79(1):77–82.
108. Kirschenbaum D, Coyle MP Jr, Leddy JP, Katsaros P, Tan F Jr, Cody RP. Shoulder strength with rotator cuff tears. Pre- and postoperative analysis. Clin Orthop Relat Res. 1993;288:174–8.
109. Rokito AS, Zuckerman JD, Gallagher MA, Cuomo F. Strength after surgical repair of the rotator cuff. J Shoulder Elbow Surg. 1996;5(1):12–7.
110. Walker SW, Couch WH, Boester GA, Sprowl DW. Isokinetic strength of the shoulder after repair of a torn rotator cuff. J Bone Joint Surg Am. 1987;69(7):1041–4.
111. Rabin SI, Post M. A comparative study of clinical muscle testing and cybex evaluation after shoulder operations. Clin Orthop Relat Res. 1990;258:147–56.
112. Plotnikoff NA, MacIntyre DL. Test-retest reliability of glenohumeral internal and external rotator strength. Clin J Sport Med. 2002;12(6):367–72.
113. Edouard P, Samozino P, Julia M, Gleizes Cervera S, Vanbiervliet W, Calmels P, et al. Reliability of isokinetic assessment of shoulder-rotator strength: a systematic review of the effect of position. J Sport Rehabil. 2011;20(3):367–83.
114. Trevethan R. Sensitivity, specificity, and predictive values: foundations, pliabilities, and pitfalls in research and practice. Front Public Health. 2017;5:307.
115. Noorani A, Goldring M, Jaggi A, Gibson J, Rees J, Bateman M, et al. BESS/BOA patient care pathways: atraumatic shoulder instability. Shoulder Elbow. 2019;11(1):60–70.
116. Farber AJ, Castillo R, Clough M, Bahk M, McFarland EG. Clinical assessment of three common tests for traumatic anterior shoulder instability. J Bone Joint Surg Am. 2006;88(7):1467–74.
117. Juel NG, Natvig B. Shoulder diagnoses in secondary care, a one year cohort. BMC Musculoskelet Disord. 2014;15:89.

118. Vincent K, Leboeuf-Yde C, Gagey O. Are degenerative rotator cuff disorders a cause of shoulder pain? Comparison of prevalence of degenerative rotator cuff disease to prevalence of nontraumatic shoulder pain through three systematic and critical reviews. J Shoulder Elbow Surg. 2017;26(5):766–73.
119. Bury J, Littlewood C. Rotator cuff disorders: a survey of current (2016) UK physiotherapy practice. Shoulder Elbow. 2018;10(1):52–61.
120. Neer CS 2nd. Anterior acromioplasty for the chronic impingement syndrome in the shoulder: a preliminary report. J Bone Joint Surg Am. 1972;54(1):41–50.
121. Cools AM, Michener LA. Shoulder pain: can one label satisfy everyone and everything? Br J Sports Med. 2017;51(5):416–7.
122. Clarsen B, Bahr R, Andersson SH, Munk R, Myklebust G. Reduced glenohumeral rotation, external rotation weakness and scapular dyskinesis are risk factors for shoulder injuries among elite male handball players: a prospective cohort study. Br J Sports Med. 2014;48(17):1327–33.
123. Kawasaki T, Ota C, Urayama S, Maki N, Nagayama M, Kaketa T, et al. Incidence of and risk factors for traumatic anterior shoulder dislocation: an epidemiologic study in high-school rugby players. J Shoulder Elbow Surg. 2014;23(11):1624–30.
124. Struyf F, Nijs J, Meeus M, Roussel NA, Mottram S, Truijen S, et al. Does scapular positioning predict shoulder pain in recreational overhead athletes? Int J Sports Med. 2014;35(1):75–82.
125. Shitara H, Kobayashi T, Yamamoto A, Shimoyama D, Ichinose T, Tajika T, et al. Prospective multifactorial analysis of preseason risk factors for shoulder and elbow injuries in high school baseball pitchers. Knee Surg Sports Traumatol Arthrosc. 2017;25(10):3303–10.
126. Myers JB, Oyama S, Hibberd EE. Scapular dysfunction in high school baseball players sustaining throwing-related upper extremity injury: a prospective study. J Shoulder Elbow Surg. 2013;22(9):1154–9.
127. Andersson SH, Bahr R, Clarsen B, Myklebust G. Risk factors for overuse shoulder injuries in a mixed-sex cohort of 329 elite handball players: previous findings could not be confirmed. Br J Sports Med. 2018;52(18):1191–8.
128. Castelein B, Cools A, Parlevliet T, Cagnie B. The influence of induced shoulder muscle pain on rotator cuff and scapulothoracic muscle activity during elevation of the arm. J Shoulder Elbow Surg. 2017;26(3):497–505.
129. Sole G, Osborne H, Wassinger C. The effect of experimentally-induced subacromial pain on proprioception. Man Ther. 2015;20(1):166–70.
130. Struyf F, Lluch E, Falla D, Meeus M, Noten S, Nijs J. Influence of shoulder pain on muscle function: implications for the assessment and therapy of shoulder disorders. Eur J Appl Physiol. 2015;115(2):225–34.
131. Wang JC, Shapiro MS. Changes in acromial morphology with age. J Shoulder Elbow Surg. 1997;6(1):55–9.
132. Worland RL, Lee D, Orozco CG, SozaRex F, Keenan J. Correlation of age, acromial morphology, and rotator cuff tear pathology diagnosed by ultrasound in asymptomatic patients. J South Orthop Assoc. 2003;12(1):23–6.
133. Ketola S, Lehtinen J, Elo P, Kortelainen S, Huhtala H, Arnala I. No difference in long-term development of rotator cuff rupture and muscle volumes in impingement patients with or without decompression. Acta Orthop. 2016;87(4):351–5.
134. Beard DJ, Rees JL, Cook JA, Rombach I, Cooper C, Merritt N, et al. Arthroscopic subacromial decompression for subacromial shoulder pain (CSAW): a multicentre, pragmatic, parallel group, placebo-controlled, three-group, randomised surgical trial. Lancet. 2018;391(10118):329–38.
135. Lahdeoja T, Karjalainen T, Jokihaara J, Salamh P, Kavaja L, Agarwal A, et al. Subacromial decompression surgery for adults with shoulder pain: a systematic review with meta-analysis. Br J Sports Med. 2020;54(11):665–73.
136. Navarro-Ledesma S, Struyf F, Labajos-Manzanares MT, Fernandez-Sanchez M, Morales-Asencio JM, Luque-Suarez A. Does the acromiohumeral distance matter in chronic rotator cuff related shoulder pain? Musculoskelet Sci Pract. 2017;29:38–42.

137. Lewis J. Rotator cuff related shoulder pain: assessment, management and uncertainties. Man Ther. 2016;23:57–68.
138. Mackenzie TA, Herrington L, Horlsey I, Cools A. An evidence-based review of current perceptions with regard to the subacromial space in shoulder impingement syndromes: is it important and what influences it? Clin Biomech (Bristol, Avon). 2015;30(7):641–8.
139. Leong HT, Fu SC, He X, Oh JH, Yamamoto N, Hang S. Risk factors for rotator cuff tendinopathy: a systematic review and meta-analysis. J Rehabil Med. 2019;51(9):627–37.
140. Zuckerman JD, Rokito A. Frozen shoulder: a consensus definition. J Shoulder Elbow Surg. 2011;20(2):322–5.
141. Lubiecki M, Carr A. Frozen shoulder: past, present, and future. J Orthop Surg (Hong Kong). 2007;15(1):1–3.
142. Walmsley S, Rivett DA, Osmotherly PG. Adhesive capsulitis: establishing consensus on clinical identifiers for stage 1 using the DELPHI technique. Phys Ther. 2009;89(9):906–17.
143. Kelley MJ, Shaffer MA, Kuhn JE, Michener LA, Seitz AL, Uhl TL, et al. Shoulder pain and mobility deficits: adhesive capsulitis. J Orthop Sports Phys Ther. 2013;43(5):A1–31.
144. Requejo-Salinas N, Fernandez-Matias R, Cadogan A, Chester R, Roy JS, Struyf F, et al. Neck or shoulder? Establishing consensus for spine screening in patients with shoulder pain: an International Modified Delphi Study. Phys Ther. 2024; https://doi.org/10.1093/ptj/pzae133.
145. Requejo-Salinas N, Lewis J, Michener LA, La Touche R, Fernandez-Matias R, Tercero-Lucas J, et al. International physical therapists consensus on clinical descriptors for diagnosing rotator cuff related shoulder pain: a Delphi study. Braz J Phys Ther. 2022;26(2):100395.
146. Hegedus EJ, Goode AP, Cook CE, Michener L, Myer CA, Myer DM, et al. Which physical examination tests provide clinicians with the most value when examining the shoulder? Update of a systematic review with meta-analysis of individual tests. Br J Sports Med. 2012;46(14):964–78.
147. Hegedus EJ, Cook C, Lewis J, Wright A, Park JY. Combining orthopedic special tests to improve diagnosis of shoulder pathology. Phys Ther Sport. 2015;16(2):87–92.
148. Michener LA, Walsworth MK, Doukas WC, Murphy KP. Reliability and diagnostic accuracy of 5 physical examination tests and combination of tests for subacromial impingement. Arch Phys Med Rehabil. 2009;90(11):1898–903.
149. Frost P, Andersen JH, Lundorf E. Is supraspinatus pathology as defined by magnetic resonance imaging associated with clinical sign of shoulder impingement? J Shoulder Elbow Surg. 1999;8(6):565–8.
150. Sher JS, Uribe JW, Posada A, Murphy BJ, Zlatkin MB. Abnormal findings on magnetic resonance images of asymptomatic shoulders. J Bone Joint Surg Am. 1995;77(1):10–5.
151. Milgrom C, Mann G, Finestone A. A prevalence study of recurrent shoulder dislocations in young adults. J Shoulder Elbow Surg. 1998;7(6):621–4.
152. Girish G, Lobo LG, Jacobson JA, Morag Y, Miller B, Jamadar DA. Ultrasound of the shoulder: asymptomatic findings in men. AJR Am J Roentgenol. 2011;197(4):W713–9.
153. Navarro-Ledesma S, Struyf F, Falla D, Luque-Suarez A. Non-traumatic chronic shoulder pain is not associated with changes in rotator cuff interval tendon thickness. Clin Biomech (Bristol, Avon). 2019;63:147–52.
154. Ottenheijm RP, Cals JW, Winkens B, Weijers RE, de Bie RA, Dinant GJ. Ultrasound imaging to tailor the treatment of acute shoulder pain: a randomised controlled trial in general practice. BMJ Open. 2016;6(11):e011048.
155. Barreto RPG, Braman JP, Ludewig PM, Ribeiro LP, Camargo PR. Bilateral magnetic resonance imaging findings in individuals with unilateral shoulder pain. J Shoulder Elbow Surg. 2019;28(9):1699–706.
156. Dunn WR, Kuhn JE, Sanders R, An Q, Baumgarten KM, Bishop JY, et al. 2013 Neer Award: predictors of failure of nonoperative treatment of chronic, symptomatic, full-thickness rotator cuff tears. J Shoulder Elbow Surg. 2016;25(8):1303–11.
157. Teunis T, Lubberts B, Reilly BT, Ring D. A systematic review and pooled analysis of the prevalence of rotator cuff disease with increasing age. J Shoulder Elbow Surg. 2014;23(12):1913–21.

158. Dean BJ, Gwilym SE, Carr AJ. Why does my shoulder hurt? A review of the neuroanatomical and biochemical basis of shoulder pain. Br J Sports Med. 2013;47(17):1095–104.
159. Lewis JS, McCreesh K, Barratt E, Hegedus EJ, Sim J. Inter-rater reliability of the shoulder symptom modification procedure in people with shoulder pain. BMJ Open Sport Exerc Med. 2016;2(1):e000181.
160. Rabin A, Irrgang JJ, Fitzgerald GK, Eubanks A. The intertester reliability of the scapular assistance test. J Orthop Sports Phys Ther. 2006;36(9):653–60.
161. Tate AR, McClure PW, Kareha S, Irwin D. Effect of the scapula reposition test on shoulder impingement symptoms and elevation strength in overhead athletes. J Orthop Sports Phys Ther. 2008;38(1):4–11.
162. Khazzam M, Gates ST, Tisano BK, Kukowski N. Diagnostic accuracy of the scapular retraction test in assessing the status of the rotator cuff. Orthop J Sports Med. 2018;6(10):2325967118799308.
163. Salamh P, Lewis J. It is time to put special tests for rotator cuff-related shoulder pain out to pasture. J Orthop Sports Phys Ther. 2020;50(5):222–5.
164. Diplock B, Hing W, Marks D. The long head of biceps at the shoulder: a scoping review. BMC Musculoskelet Disord. 2023;24(1):232.
165. Martetschlager F, Zampeli F, Tauber M, Habermeyer P. Lesions of the biceps pulley: a prospective study and classification update. JSES Int. 2020;4(2):318–23.
166. Raney EB, Thankam FG, Dilisio MF, Agrawal DK. Pain and the pathogenesis of biceps tendinopathy. Am J Transl Res. 2017;9(6):2668–83.
167. Belanger V, Dupuis F, Leblond J, Roy JS. Accuracy of examination of the long head of the biceps tendon in the clinical setting: a systematic review. J Rehabil Med. 2019;51(7):479–91.
168. Ben Kibler W, Sciascia AD, Hester P, Dome D, Jacobs C. Clinical utility of traditional and new tests in the diagnosis of biceps tendon injuries and superior labrum anterior and posterior lesions in the shoulder. Am J Sports Med. 2009;37(9):1840–7.
169. Carr RM, Shishani Y, Gobezie R. How accurate are we in detecting biceps tendinopathy? Clin Sports Med. 2016;35(1):47–55.
170. Gismervik SO, Drogset JO, Granviken F, Ro M, Leivseth G. Physical examination tests of the shoulder: a systematic review and meta-analysis of diagnostic test performance. BMC Musculoskelet Disord. 2017;18(1):41.
171. Gill HS, El Rassi G, Bahk MS, Castillo RC, McFarland EG. Physical examination for partial tears of the biceps tendon. Am J Sports Med. 2007;35(8):1334–40.
172. Clavert P, Kempf JF, Wolfram-Gabel R, Kahn JL. Are there age induced morphologic variations of the superior glenoid labrum? About 100 shoulder arthroscopies. Surg Radiol Anat. 2005;27(5):385–8.
173. Lippitt S, Matsen F. Mechanisms of glenohumeral joint stability. Clin Orthop Relat Res. 1993;291:20–8.
174. Pappas AM, Goss TP, Kleinman PK. Symptomatic shoulder instability due to lesions of the glenoid labrum. Am J Sports Med. 1983;11(5):279–88.
175. Snyder SJ, Karzel RP, Del Pizzo W, Ferkel RD, Friedman MJ. SLAP lesions of the shoulder. Arthroscopy. 1990;6(4):274–9.
176. Clavert P. Glenoid labrum pathology. Orthop Traumatol Surg Res. 2015;101(1 Suppl):S19–24.
177. Wilk KE, Macrina LC, Cain EL, Dugas JR, Andrews JR. The recognition and treatment of superior labral (slap) lesions in the overhead athlete. Int J Sports Phys Ther. 2013;8(5):579–600.
178. Maffet MW, Gartsman GM, Moseley B. Superior labrum-biceps tendon complex lesions of the shoulder. Am J Sports Med. 1995;23(1):93–8.
179. Resch H, Golser K, Thoeni H, Sperner G. Arthroscopic repair of superior glenoid labral detachment (the SLAP lesion). J Shoulder Elbow Surg. 1993;2(3):147–55.
180. Burkhart SS, Morgan CD. The peel-back mechanism: its role in producing and extending posterior type II SLAP lesions and its effect on SLAP repair rehabilitation. Arthroscopy. 1998;14(6):637–40.

181. Morgan CD, Burkhart SS, Palmeri M, Gillespie M. Type II SLAP lesions: three subtypes and their relationships to superior instability and rotator cuff tears. Arthroscopy. 1998;14(6):553–65.
182. Huri G, Hyun YS, Garbis NG, McFarland EG. Treatment of superior labrum anterior posterior lesions: a literature review. Acta Orthop Traumatol Turc. 2014;48(3):290–7.
183. Schwartzberg R, Reuss BL, Burkhart BG, Butterfield M, Wu JY, McLean KW. High prevalence of superior labral tears diagnosed by mri in middle-aged patients with asymptomatic shoulders. Orthop J Sports Med. 2016;4(1):2325967115623212.
184. Jost B, Zumstein M, Pfirrmann CW, Zanetti M, Gerber C. MRI findings in throwing shoulders: abnormalities in professional handball players. Clin Orthop Relat Res. 2005;434:130–7.
185. Ilahi OA, Labbe MR, Cosculluela P. Variants of the anterosuperior glenoid labrum and associated pathology. Arthroscopy. 2002;18(8):882–6.
186. Levigne C, Garret J, Grosclaude S, Borel F, Walch G. Surgical technique arthroscopic posterior glenoidplasty for posterosuperior glenoid impingement in throwing athletes. Clin Orthop Relat Res. 2012;470(6):1571–8.
187. Munro W, Healy R. The validity and accuracy of clinical tests used to detect labral pathology of the shoulder—a systematic review. Man Ther. 2009;14(2):119–30.
188. Calvert E, Chambers GK, Regan W, Hawkins RH, Leith JM. Special physical examination tests for superior labrum anterior posterior shoulder tears are clinically limited and invalid: a diagnostic systematic review. J Clin Epidemiol. 2009;62(5):558–63.
189. Clark RC, Chandler CC, Fuqua AC, Glymph KN, Lambert GC, Rigney KJ. Use of clinical test clusters versus advanced imaging studies in the management of patients with a suspected slap tear. Int J Sports Phys Ther. 2019;14(3):345–52.
190. Littlewood C, Malliaras P, Bateman M, Stace R, May S, Walters S. The central nervous system—an additional consideration in 'rotator cuff tendinopathy' and a potential basis for understanding response to loaded therapeutic exercise. Man Ther. 2013;18(6):468–72.
191. Gotoh M, Hamada K, Yamakawa H, Nakamura M, Yamazaki H, Ueyama Y, et al. Perforation of rotator cuff increases interleukin 1beta production in the synovium of glenohumeral joint in rotator cuff diseases. J Rheumatol. 2000;27(12):2886–92.
192. Gerber C, Fuchs B, Hodler J. The results of repair of massive tears of the rotator cuff. J Bone Joint Surg Am. 2000;82(4):505–15.
193. Conaire EO, Delaney R, Ladermann A, Schwank A, Struyf F. Massive irreparable rotator cuff tears: which patients will benefit from physiotherapy exercise programs? A narrative review. Int J Environ Res Public Health. 2023;20(7):5242.
194. Mulieri P, Dunning P, Klein S, Pupello D, Frankle M. Reverse shoulder arthroplasty for the treatment of irreparable rotator cuff tear without glenohumeral arthritis. J Bone Joint Surg Am. 2010;92(15):2544–56.
195. Denard PJ, Koo SS, Murena L, Burkhart SS. Pseudoparalysis: the importance of rotator cable integrity. Orthopedics. 2012;35(9):e1353–7.
196. Bleichert S, Renaud G, MacDermid J, Watson L, Faber K, Lenssen R, et al. Rehabilitation of symptomatic atraumatic degenerative rotator cuff tears: a clinical commentary on assessment and management. J Hand Ther. 2017;30(2):125–35.
197. Miller CA, Forrester GA, Lewis JS. The validity of the lag signs in diagnosing full-thickness tears of the rotator cuff: a preliminary investigation. Arch Phys Med Rehabil. 2008;89(6):1162–8.
198. Castoldi F, Blonna D, Hertel R. External rotation lag sign revisited: accuracy for diagnosis of full thickness supraspinatus tear. J Shoulder Elbow Surg. 2009;18(4):529–34.
199. Hertel R, Ballmer FT, Lombert SM, Gerber C. Lag signs in the diagnosis of rotator cuff rupture. J Shoulder Elbow Surg. 1996;5(4):307–13.
200. Walch G, Boulahia A, Calderone S, Robinson AH. The 'dropping' and 'hornblower's' signs in evaluation of rotator-cuff tears. J Bone Joint Surg Br. 1998;80(4):624–8.
201. Jain NB, Luz J, Higgins LD, Dong Y, Warner JJ, Matzkin E, et al. The diagnostic accuracy of special tests for rotator cuff tear: the ROW cohort study. Am J Phys Med Rehabil. 2017;96(3):176–83.

202. Sansone V, Consonni O, Maiorano E, Meroni R, Goddi A. Calcific tendinopathy of the rotator cuff: the correlation between pain and imaging features in symptomatic and asymptomatic female shoulders. Skeletal Radiol. 2016;45(1):49–55.
203. Meroni R, Piscitelli D, Valerio S, Boria P, Perin C, De Vito G, et al. Ultrasonography of the shoulder: asymptomatic findings from working-age women in the general population. J Phys Ther Sci. 2017;29(7):1219–23.
204. Louwerens JK, Sierevelt IN, van Hove RP, van den Bekerom MP, van Noort A. Prevalence of calcific deposits within the rotator cuff tendons in adults with and without subacromial pain syndrome: clinical and radiologic analysis of 1219 patients. J Shoulder Elbow Surg. 2015;24(10):1588–93.
205. Sansone VC, Meroni R, Boria P, Pisani S, Maiorano E. Are occupational repetitive movements of the upper arm associated with rotator cuff calcific tendinopathies? Rheumatol Int. 2015;35(2):273–80.
206. Uhthoff HK, Loehr JW. Calcific tendinopathy of the rotator cuff: pathogenesis, diagnosis, and management. J Am Acad Orthop Surg. 1997;5(4):183–91.
207. Le Goff B, Berthelot JM, Guillot P, Glemarec J, Maugars Y. Assessment of calcific tendonitis of rotator cuff by ultrasonography: comparison between symptomatic and asymptomatic shoulders. Joint Bone Spine. 2010;77(3):258–63.
208. Chiou HJ, Hung SC, Lin SY, Wei YS, Li MJ. Correlations among mineral components, progressive calcification process and clinical symptoms of calcific tendonitis. Rheumatology (Oxford). 2010;49(3):548–55.
209. Hackett L, Millar NL, Lam P, Murrell GA. Are the symptoms of calcific tendinitis due to neoinnervation and/or neovascularization? J Bone Joint Surg Am. 2016;98(3):186–92.
210. Bayam L, Arumilli R, Horsley I, Bayam F, Herrington L, Funk L. Testing shoulder pain mapping. Pain Med. 2017;18(7):1382–93.
211. Cui Q, Milbrandt T, Millington S, Anderson M, Hurwitz S. Treatment of posttraumatic adhesive capsulitis of the ankle: a case series. Foot Ankle Int. 2005;26(8):602–6.
212. Looney CG, Raynor B, Lowe R. Adhesive capsulitis of the hip: a review. J Am Acad Orthop Surg. 2013;21(12):749–55.
213. Millar NL, Meakins A, Struyf F, Willmore E, Campbell AL, Kirwan PD, et al. Frozen shoulder. Nat Rev Dis Primers. 2022;8(1):59.
214. Bunker TD. Frozen shoulder: unravelling the enigma. Ann R Coll Surg Engl. 1997;79(3):210–3.
215. Prodromidis AD, Charalambous CP. Is there a genetic predisposition to frozen shoulder? A systematic review and meta-analysis. JBJS Rev. 2016;4(2):e4.
216. Hand C, Clipsham K, Rees JL, Carr AJ. Long-term outcome of frozen shoulder. J Shoulder Elbow Surg. 2008;17(2):231–6.
217. Pietrzak M. Adhesive capsulitis: an age related symptom of metabolic syndrome and chronic low-grade inflammation? Med Hypotheses. 2016;88:12–7.
218. Kim DH, Kim YS, Kim BS, Sung DH, Song KS, Cho CH. Is frozen shoulder completely resolved at 2 years after the onset of disease? J Orthop Sci. 2020;25(2):224–8.
219. Wong CK, Levine WN, Deo K, Kesting RS, Mercer EA, Schram GA, et al. Natural history of frozen shoulder: fact or fiction? A systematic review. Physiotherapy. 2017;103(1):40–7.
220. Candela V, Giannicola G, Passaretti D, Venditto T, Gumina S. Adhesive capsulitis of the shoulder: pain intensity and distribution. Musculoskelet Surg. 2017;101(Suppl 2):153–8.
221. Chiaramonte R, Bonfiglio M, Chisari S. A significant relationship between personality traits and adhesive capsulitis. Rev Assoc Med Bras (1992). 2020;66(2):166–73.
222. Mertens MG, Meeus M, Noten S, Verborgt O, Fransen E, Lluch Girbes E, et al. Understanding the clinical profile of patients with frozen shoulder: a longitudinal multicentre observational study. BMJ Open. 2022;12(11):e056563.
223. Struyf F, Meeus M. Current evidence on physical therapy in patients with adhesive capsulitis: what are we missing? Clin Rheumatol. 2014;33(5):593–600.
224. Sanchis MN, Lluch E, Nijs J, Struyf F, Kangasperko M. The role of central sensitization in shoulder pain: a systematic literature review. Semin Arthritis Rheum. 2015;44(6):710–6.

225. Noten S, Struyf F, Lluch E, D'Hoore M, Van Looveren E, Meeus M. Central pain processing in patients with shoulder pain: a review of the literature. Pain Pract. 2017;17(2):267–80.
226. Leroux T, Wasserstein D, Veillette C, Khoshbin A, Henry P, Chahal J, et al. Epidemiology of primary anterior shoulder dislocation requiring closed reduction in Ontario, Canada. Am J Sports Med. 2014;42(2):442–50.
227. Zacchilli MA, Owens BD. Epidemiology of shoulder dislocations presenting to emergency departments in the United States. J Bone Joint Surg Am. 2010;92(3):542–9.
228. Bernhardson AS, Murphy CP, Aman ZS, LaPrade RF, Provencher MT. A prospective analysis of patients with anterior versus posterior shoulder instability: a matched cohort examination and surgical outcome analysis of 200 patients. Am J Sports Med. 2019;47(3):682–7.
229. Woodmass JM, Lee J, Wu IT, Desai VS, Camp CL, Dahm DL, et al. Incidence of posterior shoulder instability and trends in surgical reconstruction: a 22-year population-based study. J Shoulder Elbow Surg. 2019;28(4):611–6.
230. Brownson P, Donaldson O, Fox M, Rees JL, Rangan A, Jaggi A, et al. BESS/BOA patient care pathways: traumatic anterior shoulder instability. Shoulder Elbow. 2015;7(3):214–26.
231. Beighton P. Hypermobility scoring. Br J Rheumatol. 1988;27(2):163.
232. Beighton P, Solomon L, Soskolne CL. Articular mobility in an African population. Ann Rheum Dis. 1973;32(5):413–8.
233. Cameron KL, Duffey ML, DeBerardino TM, Stoneman PD, Jones CJ, Owens BD. Association of generalized joint hypermobility with a history of glenohumeral joint instability. J Athl Train. 2010;45(3):253–8.
234. Hippensteel KJ, Brophy R, Smith MV, Wright RW. Comprehensive review of provocative and instability physical examination tests of the shoulder. J Am Acad Orthop Surg. 2019;27(11):395–404.
235. Silliman JF, Hawkins RJ. Classification and physical diagnosis of instability of the shoulder. Clin Orthop Relat Res. 1993;291:7–19.
236. Neer CS 2nd, Foster CR. Inferior capsular shift for involuntary inferior and multidirectional instability of the shoulder. A preliminary report. J Bone Joint Surg Am. 1980;62(6):897–908.
237. Watson L, Balster S, Warby SA, Sadi J, Hoy G, Pizzari T. A comprehensive rehabilitation program for posterior instability of the shoulder. J Hand Ther. 2017;30(2):182–92.
238. Dhir J, Willis M, Watson L, Somerville L, Sadi J. Evidence-based review of clinical diagnostic tests and predictive clinical tests that evaluate response to conservative rehabilitation for posterior glenohumeral instability: a systematic review. Sports Health. 2018;10(2):141–5.
239. Skjaker SA, Enger M, Engebretsen L, Brox JI, Boe B. Young men in sports are at highest risk of acromioclavicular joint injuries: a prospective cohort study. Knee Surg Sports Traumatol Arthrosc. 2021;29(7):2039–45.
240. Mazzocca AD, Arciero RA, Bicos J. Evaluation and treatment of acromioclavicular joint injuries. Am J Sports Med. 2007;35(2):316–29.
241. Pallis M, Cameron KL, Svoboda SJ, Owens BD. Epidemiology of acromioclavicular joint injury in young athletes. Am J Sports Med. 2012;40(9):2072–7.
242. Shaffer BS. Painful conditions of the acromioclavicular joint. J Am Acad Orthop Surg. 1999;7(3):176–88.
243. Gorbaty JD, Hsu JE, Gee AO. Classifications in brief: rockwood classification of acromioclavicular joint separations. Clin Orthop Relat Res. 2017;475(1):283–7.
244. Martetschlager F, Kraus N, Scheibel M, Streich J, Venjakob A, Maier D. The diagnosis and treatment of acute dislocation of the acromioclavicular joint. Dtsch Arztebl Int. 2019;116(6):89–95.
245. Gerber C, Galantay RV, Hersche O. The pattern of pain produced by irritation of the acromioclavicular joint and the subacromial space. J Shoulder Elbow Surg. 1998;7(4):352–5.
246. Chronopoulos E, Kim TK, Park HB, Ashenbrenner D, McFarland EG. Diagnostic value of physical tests for isolated chronic acromioclavicular lesions. Am J Sports Med. 2004;32(3):655–61.

247. Krill MK, Rosas S, Kwon K, Dakkak A, Nwachukwu BU, McCormick F. A concise evidence-based physical examination for diagnosis of acromioclavicular joint pathology: a systematic review. Phys Sportsmed. 2018;46(1):98–104.
248. Cadogan A, McNair P, Laslett M, Hing W. Shoulder pain in primary care: diagnostic accuracy of clinical examination tests for non-traumatic acromioclavicular joint pain. BMC Musculoskelet Disord. 2013;14:156.
249. Garcia JA, Arguello AM, Momaya AM, Ponce BA. Sternoclavicular joint instability: symptoms, diagnosis and management. Orthop Res Rev. 2020;12:75–87.
250. Van Tongel A, Karelse A, Berghs B, Van Isacker T, De Wilde L. Diagnostic value of active protraction and retraction for sternoclavicular joint pain. BMC Musculoskelet Disord. 2014;15:421.
251. Thomas M, Bidwai A, Rangan A, Rees JL, Brownson P, Tennent D, et al. Glenohumeral osteoarthritis. Shoulder Elbow. 2016;8(3):203–14.
252. Cadogan A, Laslett M, Hing WA, McNair PJ, Coates MH. A prospective study of shoulder pain in primary care: prevalence of imaged pathology and response to guided diagnostic blocks. BMC Musculoskelet Disord. 2011;12:119.
253. Harkness EF, Macfarlane GJ, Silman AJ, McBeth J. Is musculoskeletal pain more common now than 40 years ago? Two population-based cross-sectional studies. Rheumatology (Oxford). 2005;44(7):890–5.
254. Kobayashi T, Takagishi K, Shitara H, Ichinose T, Shimoyama D, Yamamoto A, et al. Prevalence of and risk factors for shoulder osteoarthritis in Japanese middle-aged and elderly populations. J Shoulder Elbow Surg. 2014;23(5):613–9.
255. Kopec JA, Rahman MM, Berthelot JM, Le Petit C, Aghajanian J, Sayre EC, et al. Descriptive epidemiology of osteoarthritis in British Columbia. Canada. J Rheumatol. 2007;34(2):386–93.
256. Ibounig T, Simons T, Launonen A, Paavola M. Glenohumeral osteoarthritis: an overview of etiology and diagnostics. Scand J Surg. 2021;110(3):441–51.
257. Kerr R, Resnick D, Pineda C, Haghighi P. Osteoarthritis of the glenohumeral joint: a radiologic-pathologic study. AJR Am J Roentgenol. 1985;144(5):967–72.
258. Martin JA, Buckwalter JA. The role of chondrocyte senescence in the pathogenesis of osteoarthritis and in limiting cartilage repair. J Bone Joint Surg Am. 2003;85-A Suppl 2:106–10.
259. Fernandez-Moreno M, Rego I, Carreira-Garcia V, Blanco FJ. Genetics in osteoarthritis. Curr Genomics. 2008;9(8):542–7.
260. Tu C, He J, Wu B, Wang W, Li Z. An extensive review regarding the adipokines in the pathogenesis and progression of osteoarthritis. Cytokine. 2019;113:1–12.
261. Thijssen E, van Caam A, van der Kraan PM. Obesity and osteoarthritis, more than just wear and tear: pivotal roles for inflamed adipose tissue and dyslipidaemia in obesity-induced osteoarthritis. Rheumatology (Oxford). 2015;54(4):588–600.
262. Sanchez-Adams J, Leddy HA, McNulty AL, O'Conor CJ, Guilak F. The mechanobiology of articular cartilage: bearing the burden of osteoarthritis. Curr Rheumatol Rep. 2014;16(10):451.
263. Carfagno DG, Ellenbecker TS. Osteoarthritis of the glenohumeral joint: nonsurgical treatment options. Phys Sportsmed. 2002;30(4):19–30.
264. Marx RG, McCarty EC, Montemurno TD, Altchek DW, Craig EV, Warren RF. Development of arthrosis following dislocation of the shoulder: a case-control study. J Shoulder Elbow Surg. 2002;11(1):1–5.
265. Lehtinen JT, Kaarela K, Belt EA, Kautiainen HJ, Kauppi MJ, Lehto MU. Incidence of glenohumeral joint involvement in seropositive rheumatoid arthritis. A 15 year endpoint study. J Rheumatol. 2000;27(2):347–50.
266. Hasan SS, Romeo AA. Nontraumatic osteonecrosis of the humeral head. J Shoulder Elbow Surg. 2002;11(3):281–98.
267. Snoddy MC, Lee DH, Kuhn JE. Charcot shoulder and elbow: a review of the literature and update on treatment. J Shoulder Elbow Surg. 2017;26(3):544–52.
268. Dieppe PA, Lohmander LS. Pathogenesis and management of pain in osteoarthritis. Lancet. 2005;365(9463):965–73.

269. Strauss EJ, Kingery MT, Klein D, Manjunath AK. The evaluation and management of suprascapular neuropathy. J Am Acad Orthop Surg. 2020;28(15):617–27.
270. Elvey RL. Physical evaluation of the peripheral nervous system in disorders of pain and dysfunction. J Hand Ther. 1997;10(2):122–9.
271. Radhakrishnan K, Litchy WJ, O'Fallon WM, Kurland LT. Epidemiology of cervical radiculopathy. A population-based study from Rochester, Minnesota, 1976 through 1990. Brain. 1994;117(Pt 2):325–35.
272. Kelsey JL, Githens PB, Walter SD, Southwick WO, Weil U, Holford TR, et al. An epidemiological study of acute prolapsed cervical intervertebral disc. J Bone Joint Surg Am. 1984;66(6):907–14.
273. van Boxem K, Joosten EA, van Kleef M, Patijn J, van Zundert J. Pulsed radiofrequency treatment for radicular pain: where do we stand and where to go? Pain Med. 2012;13(3):351–4.
274. Wong JJ, Cote P, Quesnele JJ, Stern PJ, Mior SA. The course and prognostic factors of symptomatic cervical disc herniation with radiculopathy: a systematic review of the literature. Spine J. 2014;14(8):1781–9.
275. Woods BI, Hilibrand AS. Cervical radiculopathy: epidemiology, etiology, diagnosis, and treatment. J Spinal Disord Tech. 2015;28(5):E251–9.
276. Sampath P, Bendebba M, Davis JD, Ducker T. Outcome in patients with cervical radiculopathy. Prospective, multicenter study with independent clinical review. Spine (Phila PA 1976). 1999;24(6):591–7.
277. Wainner RS, Gill H. Diagnosis and nonoperative management of cervical radiculopathy. J Orthop Sports Phys Ther. 2000;30(12):728–44.
278. Yoss RE, Corbin KB, Maccarty CS, Love JG. Significance of symptoms and signs in localization of involved root in cervical disk protrusion. Neurology. 1957;7(10):673–83.
279. Thoomes EJ, van Geest S, van der Windt DA, Falla D, Verhagen AP, Koes BW, et al. Value of physical tests in diagnosing cervical radiculopathy: a systematic review. Spine J. 2018;18(1):179–89.
280. Rubinstein SM, Pool JJ, van Tulder MW, Riphagen II, de Vet HC. A systematic review of the diagnostic accuracy of provocative tests of the neck for diagnosing cervical radiculopathy. Eur Spine J. 2007;16(3):307–19.
281. Malanga GA, Landes P, Nadler SF. Provocative tests in cervical spine examination: historical basis and scientific analyses. Pain Physician. 2003;6(2):199–205.
282. Viikari-Juntura E, Porras M, Laasonen EM. Validity of clinical tests in the diagnosis of root compression in cervical disc disease. Spine (Phila PA 1976). 1989;14(3):253–7.
283. Gumina S, Carbone S, Albino P, Gurzi M, Postacchini F. Arm Squeeze Test: a new clinical test to distinguish neck from shoulder pain. Eur Spine J. 2013;22(7):1558–63.
284. Marciniak C. Poststroke hypertonicity: upper limb assessment and treatment. Top Stroke Rehabil. 2011;18(3):179–94.
285. McLean DE. Medical complications experienced by a cohort of stroke survivors during inpatient, tertiary-level stroke rehabilitation. Arch Phys Med Rehabil. 2004;85(3):466–9.
286. Anwer S, Alghadir A. Incidence, prevalence, and risk factors of hemiplegic shoulder pain: a systematic review. Int J Environ Res Public Health. 2020;17(14):4962.
287. Lindgren I, Jonsson AC, Norrving B, Lindgren A. Shoulder pain after stroke: a prospective population-based study. Stroke. 2007;38(2):343–8.
288. Koog YH, Jin SS, Yoon K, Min BI. Interventions for hemiplegic shoulder pain: systematic review of randomised controlled trials. Disabil Rehabil. 2010;32(4):282–91.
289. Bender L, McKenna K. Hemiplegic shoulder pain: defining the problem and its management. Disabil Rehabil. 2001;23(16):698–705.
290. Aras MD, Gokkaya NK, Comert D, Kaya A, Cakci A. Shoulder pain in hemiplegia: results from a national rehabilitation hospital in Turkey. Am J Phys Med Rehabil. 2004;83(9):713–9.
291. Pan R, Zhou M, Cai H, Guo Y, Zhan L, Li M, et al. A randomized controlled trial of a modified wheelchair arm-support to reduce shoulder pain in stroke patients. Clin Rehabil. 2018;32(1):37–47.

292. Adey-Wakeling Z, Liu E, Crotty M, Leyden J, Kleinig T, Anderson CS, et al. Hemiplegic shoulder pain reduces quality of life after acute stroke: a prospective population-based study. Am J Phys Med Rehabil. 2016;95(10):758–63.
293. Poduri KR. Shoulder pain in stroke patients and its effects on rehabilitation. J Stroke Cerebrovasc Dis. 1993;3(4):261–6.
294. Yamaguchi K, Sher JS, Andersen WK, Garretson R, Uribe JW, Hechtman K, et al. Glenohumeral motion in patients with rotator cuff tears: a comparison of asymptomatic and symptomatic shoulders. J Shoulder Elbow Surg. 2000;9(1):6–11.
295. Chantraine A, Baribeault A, Uebelhart D, Gremion G. Shoulder pain and dysfunction in hemiplegia: effects of functional electrical stimulation. Arch Phys Med Rehabil. 1999;80(3):328–31.
296. Hanger HC, Whitewood P, Brown G, Ball MC, Harper J, Cox R, et al. A randomized controlled trial of strapping to prevent post-stroke shoulder pain. Clin Rehabil. 2000;14(4):370–80.
297. Gustafsson L, McKenna K. A programme of static positional stretches does not reduce hemiplegic shoulder pain or maintain shoulder range of motion—a randomized controlled trial. Clin Rehabil. 2006;20(4):277–86.
298. Andrews AW, Bohannon RW. Decreased shoulder range of motion on paretic side after stroke. Phys Ther. 1989;69(9):768–72.
299. Vuagnat H, Chantraine A. Shoulder pain in hemiplegia revisited: contribution of functional electrical stimulation and other therapies. J Rehabil Med. 2003;35(2):49–54; quiz 6.
300. Meskers CG, Koppe PA, Konijnenbelt MH, Veeger DH, Janssen TW. Kinematic alterations in the ipsilateral shoulder of patients with hemiplegia due to stroke. Am J Phys Med Rehabil. 2005;84(2):97–105.
301. Balakrishnan S, Ward AB. The diagnosis and management of adults with spasticity. Handb Clin Neurol. 2013;110:145–60.
302. Pandyan AD, Gregoric M, Barnes MP, Wood D, Van Wijck F, Burridge J, et al. Spasticity: clinical perceptions, neurological realities and meaningful measurement. Disabil Rehabil. 2005;27(1-2):2–6.
303. Burke D, Wissel J, Donnan GA. Pathophysiology of spasticity in stroke. Neurology. 2013;80(3 Suppl 2):S20–6.
304. Holmes RJ, McManus KJ, Koulouglioti C, Hale B. Risk factors for poststroke shoulder pain: a systematic review and meta-analysis. J Stroke Cerebrovasc Dis. 2020;29(6):104787.
305. Dressler D, Bhidayasiri R, Bohlega S, Chana P, Chien HF, Chung TM, et al. Defining spasticity: a new approach considering current movement disorders terminology and botulinum toxin therapy. J Neurol. 2018;265(4):856–62.
306. Welmer AK, Widen Holmqvist L, Sommerfeld DK. Location and severity of spasticity in the first 1–2 weeks and at 3 and 18 months after stroke. Eur J Neurol. 2010;17(5):720–5.
307. Hefter H, Jost WH, Reissig A, Zakine B, Bakheit AM, Wissel J. Classification of posture in poststroke upper limb spasticity: a potential decision tool for botulinum toxin A treatment? Int J Rehabil Res. 2012;35(3):227–33.
308. Urban PP, Wolf T, Uebele M, Marx JJ, Vogt T, Stoeter P, et al. Occurence and clinical predictors of spasticity after ischemic stroke. Stroke. 2010;41(9):2016–20.
309. Parsonage MJ, Turner JW. Neuralgic amyotrophy; the shoulder-girdle syndrome. Lancet. 1948;1(6513):973–8.
310. Beghi E, Kurland LT, Mulder DW, Nicolosi A. Brachial plexus neuropathy in the population of Rochester, Minnesota, 1970–1981. Ann Neurol. 1985;18(3):320–3.
311. van Alfen N, van Eijk JJ, Ennik T, Flynn SO, Nobacht IE, Groothuis JT, et al. Incidence of neuralgic amyotrophy (Parsonage Turner syndrome) in a primary care setting—a prospective cohort study. PLoS One. 2015;10(5):e0128361.
312. van Alfen N, van Engelen BG. The clinical spectrum of neuralgic amyotrophy in 246 cases. Brain. 2006;129(Pt 2):438–50.
313. Porambo ME, Sedarsky KE, Elliott EJ, Theeler BJ, Smith JK. Nivolumab-induced neuralgic amyotrophy with hourglass-like constriction of the anterior interosseous nerve. Muscle Nerve. 2019;59(6):E40–E2.

314. Ferrante MA, Wilbourn AJ. Lesion distribution among 281 patients with sporadic neuralgic amyotrophy. Muscle Nerve. 2017;55(6):858–61.
315. Seror P. Neuralgic amyotrophy. An update. Joint Bone Spine. 2017;84(2):153–8.
316. Goetsch MR, Shen J, Jones JA, Memon A, Chatham W. Neuralgic amyotrophy presenting with multifocal myonecrosis and rhabdomyolysis. Cureus. 2020;12(3):e7382.
317. van Alfen N, van der Werf SP, van Engelen BG. Long-term pain, fatigue, and impairment in neuralgic amyotrophy. Arch Phys Med Rehabil. 2009;90(3):435–9.
318. Smittenaar CR, Petersen KA, Stewart K, Moitt N. Cancer incidence and mortality projections in the UK until 2035. Br J Cancer. 2016;115(9):1147–55.
319. Chloros GD, Haar PJ, Loughran TP, Hayes CW. Imaging of glenoid labrum lesions. Clin Sports Med. 2013;32(3):361–90.
320. Roy JS, Braen C, Leblond J, Desmeules F, Dionne CE, MacDermid JC, et al. Diagnostic accuracy of ultrasonography, MRI and MR arthrography in the characterisation of rotator cuff disorders: a systematic review and meta-analysis. Br J Sports Med. 2015;49(20):1316–28.
321. Chiou HJ, Chou YH, Wu JJ, Hsu CC, Huang DY, Chang CY. Evaluation of calcific tendonitis of the rotator cuff: role of color Doppler ultrasonography. J Ultrasound Med. 2002;21(3):289–95; quiz 96–7.
322. Farin PU, Jaroma H. Sonographic findings of rotator cuff calcifications. J Ultrasound Med. 1995;14(1):7–14.
323. Papatheodorou A, Ellinas P, Takis F, Tsanis A, Maris I, Batakis N. US of the shoulder: rotator cuff and non-rotator cuff disorders. Radiographics. 2006;26(1):e23.
324. Rangan A, Goodchild L, Gibson J, Brownson P, Thomas M, Rees J, et al. Frozen shoulder. Shoulder Elbow. 2015;7(4):299–307.
325. Choi YH, Kim DH. Correlations between clinical features and MRI findings in early adhesive capsulitis of the shoulder: a retrospective observational study. BMC Musculoskelet Disord. 2020;21(1):542.
326. Do JG, Hwang JT, Yoon KJ, Lee YT. Correlation of ultrasound findings with clinical stages and impairment in adhesive capsulitis of the shoulder. Orthop J Sports Med. 2021;9(5):23259671211003675.
327. Quan GM, Carr D, Schlicht S, Powell G, Choong PF. Lessons learnt from the painful shoulder; a case series of malignant shoulder girdle tumours misdiagnosed as frozen shoulder. Int Semin Surg Oncol. 2005;2(1):2.
328. Lewis J. Frozen shoulder contracture syndrome—aetiology, diagnosis and management. Man Ther. 2015;20(1):2–9.
329. Cho CH, Hwang I, Seo JS, Choi CH, Ko SH, Park HB, et al. Reliability of the classification and treatment of dislocations of the acromioclavicular joint. J Shoulder Elbow Surg. 2014;23(5):665–70.
330. Pifer M, Ashfaq K, Maerz T, Jackson A, Baker K, Anderson K. Intra- and interdisciplinary agreement in the rating of acromioclavicular joint dislocations. Phys Sportsmed. 2013;41(4):25–32.
331. Heers G, Hedtmann A. Correlation of ultrasonographic findings to Tossy's and Rockwood's classification of acromioclavicular joint injuries. Ultrasound Med Biol. 2005;31(6):725–32.
332. Antonio GE, Cho JH, Chung CB, Trudell DJ, Resnick D, Pictorial essay. MR imaging appearance and classification of acromioclavicular joint injury. AJR Am J Roentgenol. 2003;180(4):1103–10.
333. Schaefer FK, Schaefer PJ, Brossmann J, Hilgert RE, Heller M, Jahnke T. Experimental and clinical evaluation of acromioclavicular joint structures with new scan orientations in MRI. Eur Radiol. 2006;16(7):1488–93.
334. Kavaja L, Pajarinen J, Sinisaari I, Savolainen V, Bjorkenheim JM, Haapamaki V, et al. Arthrosis of glenohumeral joint after arthroscopic Bankart repair: a long-term follow-up of 13 years. J Shoulder Elbow Surg. 2012;21(3):350–5.
335. Gill TK, Shanahan EM, Allison D, Alcorn D, Hill CL. Prevalence of abnormalities on shoulder MRI in symptomatic and asymptomatic older adults. Int J Rheum Dis. 2014;17(8):863–71.
336. Edmond SN, Keefe FJ. Validating pain communication: current state of the science. Pain. 2015;156(2):215–9.

Index

F. Struyf, *Shoulder Pain*, https://doi.org/10.1007/978-3-031-82228-5

MIX
Papier aus verantwortungsvollen Quellen
Paper from responsible sources
FSC® C105338

If you have any concerns about our products,
you can contact us on
ProductSafety@springernature.com

In case Publisher is established outside the EU,
the EU authorized representative is:
Springer Nature Customer Service Center GmbH
Europaplatz 3, 69115 Heidelberg, Germany

Printed by Libri Plureos GmbH
in Hamburg, Germany